# MASTERING CLINICAL EMERGENCY MEDICINE

Core Skills and Strategic Approaches for Fast, Effective Decision-Making

Dr. Joe J. Gaiter
Dr. Johnny S. Lewis

© 2024 Dr. Joe J. Gaiter and Dr. Johnny S. Lewis

All rights reserved. No part of this book, MASTERING CLINICAL EMERGENCY MEDICINE: Core Skills and Strategic Approaches for Fast, Effective Decision-Making, may be reproduced, distributed, or transmitted in any form or by any means without the prior written permission of the authors, except in the case of brief quotations in a review or scholarly citation.

About the Authors:

Dr. Joe J. Gaiter, MD
Professor of Emergency Medicine and Clinical Decision-Making, McMaster University
Dr. Joe J. Gaiter is a recognized leader in emergency medicine education, specializing in the development of evidence-based frameworks that enhance clinical decision-making. With years of teaching and clinical experience, he is dedicated to preparing healthcare providers for fast, effective patient care in emergency settings.

Dr. Johnny S. Lewis, MD
Senior Clinical Researcher in Emergency Medicine, McMaster University
Dr. Johnny S. Lewis is a senior clinical researcher focused on advancing protocols in acute care and improving clinical decision-making processes in emergency medicine. His research contributions support the

integration of strategic approaches to optimize patient outcomes in high-stakes environments.

## Acknowledgments

We extend our deepest gratitude to our colleagues and mentors at McMaster University, whose unwavering commitment to excellence in emergency medicine has inspired and enriched this work. Our heartfelt thanks go to the faculty and staff in the Department of Emergency Medicine for their support and encouragement in advancing clinical education and research.

Dr. Joe J. Gaiter would like to acknowledge his students and residents, whose enthusiasm for learning and dedication to patient care have been instrumental in shaping the educational approach presented in this book. Their commitment to mastering clinical decision-making is both motivating and humbling.

Dr. Johnny S. Lewis is grateful to his research team and collaborators, whose dedication to advancing acute care protocols and clinical strategies has provided invaluable insights. Their contributions to evidence-based practice are reflected throughout this text.

Finally, we are thankful to the healthcare professionals in emergency medicine worldwide, whose resilience and expertise continue to elevate the field. This book is dedicated to all of you who strive to make a difference in the critical moments that matter most.

Dr. Joe J. Gaiter and Dr. Johnny S. Lewis

## Preface

Emergency medicine is a field that demands precision, swift decision-making, and the capacity to manage complex cases under pressure. As the dynamics of healthcare continue to evolve, so does the need for a structured approach to clinical decision-making in high-stakes settings. MASTERING CLINICAL EMERGENCY MEDICINE: Core Skills and Strategic Approaches for Fast, Effective Decision-Making was conceived to bridge the gap between theory and practice, providing healthcare professionals with the tools to excel in the fast-paced environment of emergency medicine.

This book represents the combined expertise of two seasoned professionals in emergency medicine education and research. Dr. Joe J. Gaiter, Professor of Emergency Medicine and Clinical Decision-Making at McMaster

University, brings years of teaching experience and a focus on evidence-based frameworks that refine clinical decisions. Through his work with students, residents, and practicing clinicians, Dr. Gaiter has recognized the importance of integrating core emergency medicine skills with structured, strategic thinking to prepare clinicians for the unpredictable nature of patient presentations. His contribution to this text is grounded in his dedication to advancing emergency medicine education, ensuring that each chapter reflects not only current best practices but also a roadmap for effective and efficient clinical care.

Dr. Johnny S. Lewis, Senior Clinical Researcher in Emergency Medicine at McMaster University, contributes a research-driven perspective to this book. His expertise in acute care protocols and decision-making strategies allows him to address the complexities of emergency care from a data-informed approach. Dr. Lewis's research has emphasized the importance of innovative, patient-centered solutions that can be practically implemented in emergency settings. His sections in this book focus on translating research findings into actionable strategies, equipping practitioners with advanced tools to improve patient outcomes and manage diverse clinical scenarios effectively.

MASTERING CLINICAL EMERGENCY MEDICINE is organized to provide a comprehensive yet practical guide for healthcare providers at all levels, from medical students to seasoned practitioners. The text encompasses foundational skills, such as patient assessment and triage, while also delving into advanced strategies, including critical decision pathways and dynamic treatment protocols. Each chapter includes real-world case examples, clinical insights, and frameworks to aid in mastering the principles and techniques of emergency care. By balancing clinical knowledge with structured approaches to decision-making, this book aims to instill confidence and competence in practitioners facing complex and time-sensitive situations.

We hope this text will serve as a valuable resource for those committed to mastering the art and science of emergency medicine. Whether you are a student, resident, or experienced clinician, MASTERING CLINICAL EMERGENCY MEDICINE is designed to deepen your understanding, enhance your skills, and inspire you to approach every patient encounter with precision and purpose.

Dr. Joe J. Gaiter and Dr. Johnny S. Lewis

Acknowledgement
Preface
Table of content
List of Abbreviations

Table of content

## Chapter 1: Incision and Drainage in Emergency Medicine

1. Introduction
   - Overview of I&D as the standard treatment for abscesses
   - Indications and general guidelines

2. Indications for Incision and Drainage
   - Criteria for I&D (abscess size, accessibility, and physical exam findings)
   - Role of ultrasound and needle aspiration for diagnosis
   - Classification of abscesses by location

3. Procedure Techniques
   - Preparing the patient and setting up for I&D
   - Pain management approaches
   - Step-by-step I&D procedure, including techniques for abscess probing, drainage, and use of curved hemostats

4. Special Abscess Types
   - Hidradenitis Suppurativa
   - Pilonidal and Sebaceous Cysts
   - Perirectal Abscesses

5. Contraindications
   - Cases where I&D is not advised
   - Large or deep abscesses and requirements for anesthesia
   - Prophylactic antibiotic recommendations for endocarditis risk patients

6. Equipment Needed
   - List of essential tools

- Iodoform gauze packing and irrigation materials

7. Detailed Procedure
    - Preparation and Consent
    - Anesthetic Administration
    - Incision and Drainage
    - Wound Packing and Dressing

8. Special Techniques for Bartholin Gland Abscess
    - Use of Word catheter insertion to maintain drainage and promote fistula formation
    - Instructions for follow-up after 48 hours

9. Complications
    - Risks of scarring, nerve injury, and transient bacteremia
    - Guidelines for managing potential adverse outcomes

## Chapter 2: Arterial Blood Gas Analysis – Key Clinical Guidelines

1. Overview
   - Importance of ABG analysis in emergency settings
   - Assessment of respiratory and metabolic status

2. Indications for ABG
   - Primary indications
   - Secondary indication
   - Situations where arterial blood may substitute venous sampling

3. Contraindications
   - Conditions to approach with caution
   - Vascular considerations
   - Allen test as a tool for assessing collateral circulation

4. Required Equipment
   - Essential tools
   - Optional tools

5. Procedure Steps
   - Pre-Procedure
   - Arterial Location
   - Needle Insertion
   - Post-Procedure Care

6. Complications
   - Possible risks
   - Mitigation strategies for safer ABG collection

## Chapter 3: Central Venous Access

1. Overview
   - Importance of central venous access in emergency settings
   - Site selection considerations for optimal access

2. Indications for Central Venous Access
   - Critical resuscitation in trauma and medical patients
   - Use cases

- Indications for patients with difficult peripheral access

3. Contraindications
   - Situations where peripheral access is preferable
   - Local contraindications
   - Patient-specific consideration

4. Required Equipment
   - Overview of central line kits and essential components
   - Types of central lines

5. Procedure Steps
   - Preparation
   - Technique
   - Insertion of needle and guidewire
   - Step-by-step catheter placement
   - Guidewire removal and placement confirmation

6. Site-Specific Techniques
   - Internal Jugular Cannulation

- Subclavian Cannulation
- Femoral Vein Cannulation

7. Complications

    - General complications
    - Site-specific risks
    - Internal Jugular
    - Subclavian
    - Femoral

**Chapter 4: Procedural Sedation**

1. Introduction to Procedural Sedation
    - Definition and Importance
    - Goals of Procedural Sedation
    - Key Points for Safety and Efficacy

2. Indications for Procedural Sedation
    - Clinical Situations for Sedation Use
    - Sedation Agents and Their Categories
    - Patient Evaluation and Suitability

3. Contraindications and Risk Assessment

- Absolute and Relative Contraindications
- High-Risk Conditions Requiring Specialist Consultation

4. Required Equipment and Monitoring
    - Essential Monitoring Tools and Equipment Setup
    - Pre-Procedure Preparation for Patient Safety

5. Procedure for Sedation
    - Pre-Procedure Assessment and Informed Consent
    - Medication Selection and Administration Techniques
    - Monitoring During Procedure and Patient Observation

6. Common Medications Used in Procedural Sedation
    - Overview of Sedatives, Analgesics, and Dissociative Agents

- Detailed Dosages, Effects, and Reversal Agents

7. Reversal Agents
   - Flumazenil for Benzodiazepines
   - Naloxone for Opioids

8. Complications and Management
   - Respiratory Depression and Airway Complications
   - Nausea, Vomiting, and Aspiration Risks
   - Inadequate or Prolonged Sedation

## Chapter 5: Lumbar Puncture

1. Introduction
   - Overview of lumbar puncture (LP) and its clinical applications.

2. Indications
   - Diagnostic uses
   - Therapeutic uses

3. Contraindications
    - Absolute
    - Relative

4. Pre-Procedure Preparation
    - Anatomical landmarks and sterile technique.
    - Imaging requirements

5. Equipment and Supplies
    - LP kit components
    - Imaging support

6. Procedure Technique
    - Positioning and needle insertion steps.
    - Use of a manometer for CSF pressure measurement.
    - Tube collection and sample management.

7. Complications
    - Common
    - Rare but serious

- Traumatic tap and differentiation from SAH.

8. Post-Procedure Management
    - Headache management
    - Monitoring for infection and neurological complications.

9. Summary
    - Key points for safe and effective LP execution.

## Chapter 6: Laceration Repair

1. Introduction
    - Optimal Timing for Wound Closure
    - Foreign Body Removal Priorities

2. Indications for Laceration Repair
    - Criteria for Wound Closure
    - Closure Methods

3. Contraindications

- Patient-Related Factors
- Wound-Related Factors

4. Special Considerations
   - Blunt vs. Sharp Injuries
   - High-Risk Wounds
   - Limitations of Staples and Tissue Adhesive

5. Required Equipment
   - Essential Supplies and Instruments
   - Suture Recommendations for Different Body Areas

6. Procedure Overview
   - Timing of Closure
   - Wound Preparation
   - Wound Closure Techniques

7. Aftercare and Wound Management
   - Moisture and Antibiotics
   - Tetanus Prophylaxis Guidelines
   - Dressing and Covering the Wound

## Chapter 7: Needle and Tube Thoracostomy: Key Guidelines and Procedure

1. Introduction
    - Key Points
    - Safety Note on Rib Positioning and Pulmonary Blebs

2. Indications
    - Needle Thoracostomy for Tension Pneumothorax
    - Tube Thoracostomy for Pneumothorax, Hemothorax, and Large Pleural Effusions

3. Contraindications
    - Differentiating Pulmonary Blebs/Bullae from Pneumothorax
    - Alternatives to Tube Thoracostomy

4. Required Equipment
    - Needle Thoracostomy Equipment

- Tube Thoracostomy Equipment by Age and Condition

5. Procedure
    - Needle Thoracostomy
    - Tube Thoracostomy

6. Complications
    - Needle Thoracostomy Complications
    - Decompression Failure and Body Habitus Considerations
    - Tube Thoracostomy Complications
    - Infection, Tube Displacement, and Bleeding
    - Improper Placement and Reexpansion Pulmonary Edema Management

**Chapter 8: Introduction to Emergency Ultrasonography**

1. Introduction
    - Key Points

2. Indications

- Core Applications of EUS

3. Contraindications
    - Limitations of EUS Due to Patient Factors or Physician Expertise
    - When to Consider Additional Imaging

4. Equipment
    - Basics of EUS Technology and Image Formation
    - Frequency: Superficial vs. Deep Imaging
    - Echogenicity
    - Orientation

5. Ultrasound Modes
    - Brightness (B) Mode, Motion (M) Mode, and Doppler Modes

6. Procedure
    - Basic FAST Examination Technique and Views

7. Complications

- Image Clarity Issues and Misinterpretation Risks

## Chapter 9: Emergency Medical Services

1. Introduction

    - Overview of EMS

2. Workforce
    - EMS Staffing in Urban, Suburban, and Rural Areas

3. Training
    - Certification Levels

4. Communications and Access to Care
    - Role of the "911" System and Dispatcher Responsibilities

5. Transportation

    - Types of EMS Vehicles
    - Air Transport Options

6. Critical Care Facilities
    - Selecting Patient Destinations and Use of Specialty Centers

7. Public Safety Coordination
    - Collaboration Among Police, Fire, and EMS Services

8. Community Involvement
    - Public Education, CPR Training, and Community Engagement

9. Patient Transfer and Documentation
    - Inter-Facility Transfers and Documentation Challenges

10. Quality Control and Disaster Preparedness
    - Continuous Quality Improvement and Disaster Response Protocols

11. Mutual Aid

- Interagency Agreements and Coordinated Emergency Responses

**Chapter 10: Cardiopulmonary Arrest**

1. Introduction
    - Overview of Cardiopulmonary Arrest and Sudden Cardiac Death (SCD)
    - Key Risk Factors and Survival Statistics

2. Clinical Evaluation and Diagnostic Approach
    - History
    - Physical Examination
    - Diagnostic Studies

3. Procedures
    - Pericardiocentesis for Cardiac Tamponade
    - Needle Thoracostomy for Tension Pneumothorax

4. Management and Treatment

- Defibrillation
- Chest Compressions
- Airway Management
- Pharmacologic Intervention

5. Post-Resuscitation Care
   - Therapeutic Hypothermia and Rewarming Protocol

6. Disposition
   - ICU/Critical Care Admission and Evaluation for Underlying Causes

## Chapter 11: Airway Management - Key Insights and Evidence-Based Practice

1. Introduction
   - Importance of Airway Management
   - Indicators for Intubation and Decision-Making

2. Clinical Approach to Airway Management
   - Criteria for Intubation
   - Airway Protection

- Oxygenation and Ventilation Failure
- Alternative Measures

3. Techniques and Equipment Selection
    - Bag-Valve-Mask (BVM) Ventilation
    - Rapid Sequence Intubation (RSI)
    - Selection of Equipment and Endotracheal Tubes (ETT)

4. Clinical Presentation
    - History
    - Physical Examination

5. Diagnostic Studies
    - Blood Gas Analysis and Pulse Oximetry
    - Chest X-Ray for ETT Placement Verification

6. Medical Decision-Making
    - Identifying Reversible Causes of Airway Compromise
    - Assessing for Difficult Airway and Adapting Techniques

7. Procedures
    - Bag-Valve-Mask Ventilation
    - Rapid Sequence Intubation

## Chapter 12: Shock Management in Clinical Practice

1. Introduction
    - Overview and Statistics
    - Types of Shock

2. Pathophysiology of Shock
    - Phases of Shock Progression
    - Autonomic Response
    - Cellular Hypoxia
    - Inflammatory Cascade

3. Clinical Presentation
    - History and Physical Examination
    - Distinguishing Features by Shock Type

4. Diagnostic Workup

- Laboratory Tests
- Key Indicators
- Imaging Modalities
- Chest X-ray, Ultrasound, CT Scans

5. Procedures and Medical Decision Making
   - Intubation and Central Line Placement
   - Rapid Identification and Treatment

6. Treatment Strategies by Shock Type
   - General Measures
   - Specific Interventions
   - Hypovolemic, Distributive, Obstructive Shock

## Chapter 13: Chest Pain Evaluation and Management

1. Introduction
   - Epidemiology and Importance of Systematic Approach
   - Somatic vs. Visceral Pain

2. Clinical Presentation
    - History and Pain Characteristics
    - Location, Radiation, Duration, Associated Symptoms
    - Physical Examination
    - Key Findings by Condition

3. Diagnostic Studies
    - ECG and Cardiac Markers
    - Imaging
    - Chest X-ray, CT Angiography, Echocardiography

4. Medical Decision Making
    - Integration of Clinical Data
    - Pre-Test Probability and Risk Assessment

5. Treatment
    - Acute Coronary Syndrome (ACS)
    - Aortic Dissection, Pulmonary Embolism, Boerhaave Syndrome
    - Pneumothorax, Pericardial Tamponade

7. Disposition
   - Criteria for Admission
   - Guidelines for Safe Discharge

## Chapter 14: Acute Coronary Syndromes (ACS)

1. Introduction
   - Definition and epidemiology
   - Pathophysiology of ACS and plaque rupture mechanisms

2. Classification of ACS
   - Unstable Angina (UA)
   - Non-ST-Segment Elevation Myocardial Infarction (NSTEMI)
   - ST-Segment Elevation Myocardial Infarction (STEMI)

3. Coronary Artery Anatomy
   - Overview of coronary artery structure
   - Importance in ACS management and ECG interpretation

4. Risk Factors
    - Age, gender, lifestyle, and comorbidities in CAD risk

5. Clinical Presentation
    - History and symptomatology, including atypical presentations
    - Physical examination and vital signs

6. Diagnostic Studies
    - Electrocardiogram (ECG) patterns in ACS
    - ST-segment elevation and depression
    - T-wave abnormalities
    - Q-waves
    - Anatomical ECG considerations for MI localization

7. Laboratory Analysis
    - Cardiac biomarkers
    - Timing and interpretation of marker elevation

8. Imaging
    - Role of chest X-ray in differential diagnosis

9. Medical Decision Making
    - Immediate ECG and risk stratification
    - Sequential ECGs and cardiac marker testing

10. Treatment
    - Initial stabilization
    - Medications
    - Nitroglycerin
    - Morphine
    - Antiplatelet Therapy
    - Glycoprotein IIb/IIIa inhibitors
    - Anticoagulation
    - Beta-blockers
    - Reperfusion Therapy

11. Disposition
    - Criteria for admission and critical care transfer

- Discharge considerations for low-risk patients

## Chapter 15: Congestive Heart Failure (CHF)

1. Introduction
   - Overview of CHF prevalence and impact
   - Common causes and classification

2. Pathophysiology of Acute Decompensated CHF
   - Mechanisms leading to pulmonary edema and respiratory distress
   - Systemic vascular resistance and its effects on myocardial function

3. Precipitants of Decompensated CHF
   - Common and additional causes

4. Clinical Presentation
   - Symptom assessment

- Signs of pulmonary and systemic congestion

5. Physical Examination
    - Rapid assessment for stability and respiratory distress
    - Identification of left and right ventricular failure signs

6. Diagnostic Studies
    - Laboratory Studies
    - ECG: Identification of injury and arrhythmias
    - Imaging: Chest X-ray and echocardiography for CHF assessment

7. Medical Decision-Making
    - Assessment and intervention for respiratory distress
    - Role of inotropic and vasopressor support in hypotensive patients

8. Treatment

- Goals of therapy
- Treatment steps based on severity

9. Medications for CHF Management
    - Vasodilators
    - Loop Diuretics
    - Inotropes and Pressors

10. General Considerations
    - Blood pressure monitoring during treatment
    - Duration of use and safety notes for CHF medications

## Chapter 16: Dysrhythmias

1. Introduction
    - Importance of dysrhythmia recognition
    - Classification by rate
    - Overview of cardiac conduction and rhythm

2. ECG Considerations

- Performing and interpreting a 12-lead ECG
- Identifying underlying causes

3. ECG Components
   - Analysis of P wave, QRS complex, and T wave
   - Characteristics of normal vs. abnormal conduction

4. Classification of Dysrhythmias
   - Narrow vs. wide QRS complexes
   - Detailed rhythm classification

5. Clinical Presentation
   - History and examination in stable vs. unstable cases

6. Diagnostic Studies
   - Laboratory and imaging workup
   - ECG and rhythm strip analysis

7. Bradydysrhythmias
   - Assessment and types

- Treatment approach for Mobitz Type I/II and third-degree blocks

8. Tachydysrhythmias
   - Differentiation of rhythms
   - Management strategies based on stability and QRS width

9. Management of Wide-Complex Tachycardias
   - Protocol for ventricular tachycardia and torsades de pointes

10. Treatment Approaches
    - Airway, breathing, circulation (ABCs)
    - Medications and interventions by rhythm type

11. Disposition
    - Admission criteria for monitoring and discharge guidelines

## Chapter 17: Aortic Dissection

1. Introduction
   - Epidemiology and demographic risk factors
   - Pathophysiology of aortic dissection

2. Clinical Presentation
   - Recognizing symptoms

3. Risk Factors
   - Connective tissue disorders and genetic predispositions

4. Physical Examination
   - Vital signs and differential findings

5. Diagnostic Studies
   - Role of imaging
   - Laboratory tests for ruling out other causes

6. Management
   - Hemodynamic stabilization and initial pharmacologic management

- Surgical vs. medical treatment decisions

8. Complications
   - Potential outcomes and associated risks

9. Disposition and Follow-up
   - Criteria for ICU admission
   - Long-term management and surveillance


## Chapter 18: Hypertensive Emergencies: Summary and Analysis

1. Introduction
   - Prevalence of Hypertension
   - Classification
   - Pathophysiology of Hypertensive Emergencies

2. Clinical Presentation
   - History and Symptoms

- Specific Conditions

3. Physical Examination
    - Accurate BP Measurement
    - Neurological, Cardiac, Pulmonary, and Abdominal Assessments

4. Diagnostic Studies
    - ECG and Laboratory Tests
    - Imaging Studies

5. Medical Decision Making
    - Identification of Hypertensive Emergencies
    - Diagnostic Confirmation and Treatment Approach

6. Treatment
    - BP Control and Medication Choices
    - Specific Management for Aortic Dissection and Intracranial Hemorrhage

**Chapter 19: Syncope Management**

1. Introduction
    - Definition and Epidemiology of Syncope
    - Causes: Neural-mediated, Orthostatic, Cerebrovascular, and Cardiac

3. Clinical Presentation
    - History: Identifying Warning Symptoms
    - Physical Examination and Findings

4. Diagnostic Studies
    - Laboratory Tests
    - ECG and Imaging

5. Medical Decision Making
    - Structured Approach to Differential Diagnosis
    - Prioritization of Life-threatening Causes

6. Treatment

- Supportive Care and Specific Management Strategies
- Cardiac Syncope: ACLS Guidelines
- Cerebrovascular Syncope
- Orthostatic Syncope
- Reflex/Vasovagal Syncope

7. Disposition
   - Admission Criteria for Cardiac Syncope
   - Discharge Criteria for Low-Risk Patients

## Chapter 20: Dyspnea - An Overview of Assessment and Management

1. Introduction
   - Definition and clinical perspective
   - Mechanisms of dyspnea
   - Immediate treatment in severe respiratory distress

2. Clinical Presentation

- Three critical questions:

3. History Taking
    - Exertional Dyspnea
    - Positional Dyspnea
    - Transient and Recurrent Dyspnea

4. Physical Examination
    - Visual appearance and signs of respiratory distress
    - Anatomical assessment:

5. Cardiac Considerations
    - Role of cardiac dysfunction in dyspnea
    - Cardiac examination findings and diagnostics

7. Hemoglobin and Blood Volume
    - Impact of anemia and blood volume on dyspnea
    - Monitoring and management

## List of Abbreviations

1. **ACLS** – Advanced Cardiovascular Life Support

2. **BLS** – Basic Life Support

3. **CPT** – Current Procedural Terminology

4. **CT** – Computed Tomography

5. **ECG** – Electrocardiogram

6. **EMT** – Emergency Medical Technician

7. **ETT** – Endotracheal Tube

8. **ICU** – Intensive Care Unit

9. **IV** – Intravenous

10. **KIA** – Killed in Action (military context for emergency care)

11. **LBW** – Low Birth Weight

12. **PE** – Pulmonary Embolism

13. **PALS** – Pediatric Advanced Life Support

14. **PRBC** – Packed Red Blood Cells

15. **SATS** – Oxygen Saturation Levels

16. **STEMI** – ST-Elevation Myocardial Infarction

17. **TBI** – Traumatic Brain Injury

18. **TIA** – Transient Ischemic Attack

19. **TIA** – Trauma-Informed Assessment

20. **V-Fib** – Ventricular Fibrillation

21. **VT** – Ventricular Tachycardia

22. **WBC** – White Blood Cells

# Chapter 1
## Incision and Drainage in Emergency Medicine

### Key Points

Preferred Procedure: Incision and drainage (I&D) is the optimal treatment for subcutaneous abscesses.

Antibiotics: These are not typically needed unless cellulitis is also present.

### Indications

I&D is the primary treatment for subcutaneous abscesses. Abscesses greater than 5 mm that can be accessed through the skin should be drained. Antibiotics alone are insufficient for treating abscesses, and antibiotics are generally unnecessary if there is no associated cellulitis after drainage.

Physical examination reveals abscesses through swelling, pain, redness, and fluctuance. Some abscesses may drain on their own, confirming the diagnosis. Ultrasound can assist by highlighting fluid beneath the skin, and needle aspiration can verify pus presence.

Abscesses have various designations based on location. For example, paronychia involves infection around the nail, while felons involve the volar pad of the finger, needing specialized drainage. Bartholin gland abscesses occur when ducts in the vaginal vestibule are blocked; I&D with a Word catheter is often used to maintain drainage. In severe cases, gland removal may prevent recurrence.

Procedure Tips: Use a curved hemostat to probe and disrupt abscess pockets and reveal any deeper tracks.

Pain Management: Local anesthesia may be challenging, potentially requiring a field block, analgesics, or sedation.

Hidradenitis suppurativa—a recurring condition of the apocrine glands, often in the axilla or groin—can lead to multiple abscesses, treated with I&D in the emergency setting. I&D also treats infected pilonidal or sebaceous cysts, although subsequent surgical removal of the cyst capsule may be necessary to prevent recurrence.

Perirectal abscesses include superficial types (perianal), manageable by emergency physicians, and deeper types (e.g., ischiorectal, intersphincteric), which require surgical drainage. Perianal abscesses manifest as painful, fluctuant masses near the anus, while deeper abscesses present with rectal pain, defecation pain, and possible systemic symptoms like fever.

Contraindications

I&D should not be performed if cellulitis is present without an abscess. Pulsatile masses, which could be infected pseudoaneurysms, must not be incised. Large or deep abscesses may require drainage under anesthesia, and patients at risk for endocarditis should receive prophylactic antibiotics.

Equipment

Essential equipment includes:

Skin cleansers (e.g., povidone-iodine or chlorhexidine)

Anesthetics (1% lidocaine or 0.25% bupivacaine with epinephrine)

Syringes and needles for anesthetic administration

Protective gear (gloves, gown, face shield)

11-blade scalpel

Curved hemostat

Iodoform gauze for packing

30 mL syringe with saline for irrigation

Procedure

Before the procedure, discuss risks and benefits with the patient and obtain consent. Confirm the abscess location, if necessary, with ultrasound. Wash hands and use universal precautions (gloves, gown, face shield). Position the patient for optimal access and cleanse the area.

Inject anesthetic just beneath the dermis around the abscess site without directly injecting into the abscess cavity to avoid increasing pressure and pain. For larger abscesses, additional anesthesia or sedation may be necessary. If abscess presence is uncertain, use a syringe with an 18- or 20-gauge needle to attempt aspiration of pus.

With a scalpel, make a single incision at the point of greatest fluctuance, oriented along the abscess's long axis. Incise approximately two-thirds the diameter of the abscess cavity. Apply gentle pressure to express pus, and use a hemostat to break up any internal loculations and identify deeper tracks. Consider obtaining a wound culture.

Gently irrigate until clear, then pack the wound with iodoform gauze to facilitate ongoing drainage. Cover the site with gauze.

When treating a Bartholin gland abscess, insert a Word catheter in the opening to allow continued drainage and fistula formation. The patient should return in 48 hours for packing removal. If pus and symptoms have resolved, healing can proceed by secondary intention.

Complications

Potential complications include scarring, cutaneous nerve injury, and transient bacteremia.

Suggested Reading

1. Fitch MT, Manthey DE, McGinnis HD, et al. Abscess incision and drainage. N Engl J Med. 2007;357:e20.

2. Hankin A, Everett WW. Are antibiotics necessary after incision and drainage of a cutaneous abscess? Ann Emerg Med. 2007;50:49-51.

3. Kelly EW, Magilner D. Soft tissue infections. In: Tintinalli JE, et al. Tintinalli's Emergency Medicine: A Comprehensive Study Guide. 7th ed. New York: McGraw-Hill; 2011:1014-1024.

## Chapter 2
## Arterial Blood Gas Analysis: Key Clinical Guidelines

Overview

Arterial blood gas (ABG) analysis, often performed through arterial puncture, is a critical diagnostic tool in emergency medicine, particularly for assessing respiratory and metabolic status. This analysis enables rapid quantification of oxygen and carbon dioxide levels, along with pH, which are essential in managing patients with respiratory or metabolic issues.

Indications

ABG is primarily indicated for evaluating a patient's oxygen and carbon dioxide levels, as well as blood pH. Secondary uses include measuring levels of carboxyhemoglobin, methemoglobin, and basic electrolytes, which can vary depending on laboratory capabilities. In specific cases, such as patients with limited venous access due to obesity or a history of intravenous drug use, arterial blood can serve as an alternative for routine testing when venous sampling is not feasible.

Contraindications

While few absolute contraindications exist, specific situations warrant caution. Contraindications include trauma, infection, or compromised skin integrity at the puncture site, as these could increase the risk of infection or vascular damage. Patients on anticoagulants or with coagulopathies are at an elevated risk of bleeding, hematoma, or rare complications like compartment syndrome. Additionally, prior vascular surgeries or inadequate blood flow, particularly in the palmar arch, present risks. The Allen test, traditionally used to assess collateral circulation, may guide site selection, although its routine necessity remains debated.

Required Equipment

Common equipment for ABG collection includes:

Alcohol, chlorhexidine, or iodine wipes for skin disinfection

A heparinized syringe (2-3 mL) with a fine needle (23-25 gauge)

Syringe cap for specimen handling

Personal protective gear

Gauze for post-procedure dressing

Optional items include lidocaine for local anesthesia, ultrasound guidance if needed, and ice for samples requiring extended processing time.

Procedure

The procedure often begins with the Allen test to evaluate blood flow adequacy. For this, both the radial and ulnar arteries are occluded while the patient clenches their fist, followed by the release of the ulnar artery, with rapid color return suggesting adequate collateral circulation.

To locate the radial artery, palpate it at the wrist's proximal crease, between the radius and flexor carpi radialis tendon. Position the wrist to improve accessibility, often using a rolled towel. After disinfecting and anesthetizing the skin, locate the artery by pulse, and insert the needle at a 30-45 degree angle. Blood should flow passively into the syringe once the artery is accessed. Adjustments to the needle's position are sometimes necessary; however, moving the needle in a deeper arc is avoided to prevent vascular injury. Once sufficient blood is obtained, maintain pressure on the site for five minutes to minimize hematoma risk.

Complications

While ABG sampling is generally safe, potential complications include infection, bleeding, arterial damage, pseudoaneurysm, and nerve injury.

Further Reading

1. Dev et al., Arterial Puncture for Blood Gas Analysis (N Engl J Med, 2011)

2. Giner et al., Pain during Arterial Puncture (Chest, 1996)

3. Haji Seyed Javadi et al., Lidocaine Jet Injection for ABG Pain Reduction (Am J Emerg Med, 2012)

4. Haynes & Mitchell, Ultrasound-Guided Arterial Puncture (Resp Care, 2010)

5. Shiver et al., Ultrasound vs Blind Radial Arterial Catheter Placement (Acad Emerg Med, 2006)

# Chapter 3
# Central Venous Access

## Key Points

Proficiency in central venous access is critical for emergency physicians, as it often becomes necessary in life-threatening situations.

Central venous access can be achieved through multiple routes above or below the diaphragm. Selection of the access site should consider both the clinical need and the patient's body habitus or trauma pattern.

While the complication rate for experienced practitioners is generally low, serious adverse events can occur.

## Indications for Central Venous Access

In the emergency department (ED), central venous catheter placement is primarily indicated for resuscitating critically ill or trauma patients. Medical patients may require central access for large-volume fluid resuscitation, central venous pressure monitoring, administration of medications (e.g., hypertonic saline or parenteral nutrition) that may harm peripheral veins, transvenous pacing, or emergency dialysis. Trauma patients often require central venous access for rapid resuscitation with fluids or blood. Additionally, central access is valuable in patients where peripheral IV access proves challenging.

Contraindications

Central venous access should be avoided when peripheral access is feasible, or if specific contraindications exist. Local site contraindications include overlying cellulitis or structural abnormalities, such as significant trauma, that distort anatomic landmarks. Patients with known coagulopathy should not undergo subclavian vein cannulation (due to the non-compressible nature of the site) and have relative contraindications for jugular and femoral access. Patient cooperation, or the ability to remain still, is also crucial; sedation may be required if a patient is uncooperative.

Required Equipment

Central venous cannulation typically requires a pre-packaged central line kit, which includes essential items such as povidone-iodine swabs, introducer needle, J-tip guidewire, syringes, lidocaine, scalpel, dilator, central line catheter, and sutures. There are two main types of central lines used in the ED:

Triple-lumen catheters: Useful for patients needing multiple medications or when peripheral access is difficult.

Sheath introducer (Cordis) catheters: Wider and shorter, used for procedures requiring rapid fluid infusion or pacemaker introduction, with flow rates up to 1 liter per minute.

Procedure

Before beginning, explain the risks and benefits to the patient or their representative, and obtain informed consent unless the procedure is emergent. Following technique:

1. Use a large-bore needle with a syringe to access the vein; ensure there is free, non-pulsatile blood flow.

2. Insert the guidewire through the needle, withdrawing and reinserting if resistance is encountered.

3. Remove the needle while securely holding the guidewire.

4. Make a superficial incision at the guidewire entry site.

5. Advance the dilator (and catheter for Cordis) over the guidewire into the vessel.

6. Remove the dilator and thread the catheter over the wire.

7. Securely advance the catheter into the vein, remove the guidewire, and confirm catheter placement by aspirating blood.

Internal Jugular Cannulation: Position the patient in slight Trendelenburg with the head rotated to the opposite side. Identify the triangle formed by the sternocleidomastoid muscle heads and palpate the carotid artery pulse. Insert the needle at the triangle apex toward the ipsilateral nipple.

Subclavian Cannulation: Position the patient supine, with the shoulders retracted. Insert the needle inferior to the clavicle at the junction of its medial and middle thirds, directing it toward the suprasternal notch.

Femoral Vein Cannulation: Position the needle at a 45-degree angle just medial to the femoral artery pulse. In pulseless patients, use the inguinal ligament landmarks for needle placement.

Complications

Complications can arise across all access sites, including infection, bleeding, vessel or arterial injury, and air embolism. Specific risks vary by site:

Internal Jugular: Potential for airway compression from hematoma, carotid artery dissection, pneumothorax, and arrhythmias.

Subclavian: Risk of pneumothorax and arrhythmias.

Femoral: Increased risk of deep vein thrombosis, retroperitoneal bleeding, and bowel perforation.

# Chapter 4
## Procedural Sedation: Overview and Guidelines

Key Points:

Procedural sedation involves administering analgesic and sedative agents to induce a depressed level of consciousness, enabling the performance of medical procedures without patient movement or memory.

The primary goals of procedural sedation are to achieve analgesia (pain relief), amnesia (memory loss), and anxiolysis (anxiety reduction) during potentially painful or distressing procedures.

Sedation should maintain cardiorespiratory function without the need for advanced airway support.

Proper pre-procedure assessment, medication selection, and equipment readiness are crucial to ensure patient safety.

Indications

Procedural sedation is used to reduce a patient's awareness while maintaining their protective airway reflexes and the ability to breathe spontaneously. This technique is employed in various clinical situations that may cause pain or anxiety, such as joint reduction, lumbar punctures, pediatric radiological procedures, incision and drainage, or cardioversion. Sedation helps patients remain calm and still during procedures while minimizing discomfort.

The medications used in procedural sedation typically fall into three categories: sedatives, analgesics, and dissociative agents. The use of these medications is common and generally considered safe in emergency settings. Before sedation, the patient's medical history should be assessed, particularly regarding systemic diseases and the potential for a difficult airway. The American Society of Anesthesiologists (ASA) physical status classification is used to evaluate a patient's suitability for sedation.

For patients classified as ASA I or II (healthy patients or those with mild systemic disease), the risk of complications from procedural sedation is low, generally less than 5%.

Contraindications

Certain conditions make procedural sedation unsuitable. These include:

ASA class III or IV patients (those with severe systemic diseases or conditions that pose a constant threat to life).

Altered mental status or hemodynamic instability.

Known allergies to sedation agents.

Lack of necessary equipment or qualified personnel.

In addition, oral intake within three hours prior to sedation is a relative contraindication due to the risk of aspiration. High-risk cases may require consultation with anesthesia specialists or sedation in an operating room setting.

Equipment

Effective monitoring and equipment are essential to prevent complications, particularly respiratory depression. Key monitoring tools include continuous pulse oximetry, cardiac monitoring, and end-tidal $CO_2$ capnography (if available). An IV access point, oxygen delivery system, suction, and airway management tools (such as bag-valve-mask, supraglottic airway, and intubation equipment) should all be prepared. Personnel should be well-trained in airway management and patient monitoring.

Procedure

Pre-procedure preparation involves gathering a complete medical history, checking for allergies or adverse reactions to anesthetic agents, and evaluating the patient's physical condition, particularly airway considerations. For example, factors like neck mobility, obesity, and the Mallampati classification (which assesses the difficulty of intubation) should be taken into account. Sedation is generally reserved for ASA class I and II patients, with a fasting period of at least three hours before the procedure. However, some studies suggest that shorter fasting periods do not significantly increase the risk of aspiration.

Informed consent must be obtained and documented. Medication administration should be based on the procedure type and patient response. Commonly used sedation combinations include midazolam with fentanyl, or ketamine alone or with atropine (for pediatric patients). Propofol combined with fentanyl or midazolam with analgesics are also frequently used regimens.

The physician performs the procedure while monitoring personnel assess the patient's status. Post-procedure, the patient should be observed until they return to baseline mental function and stable vital signs. Discharge criteria include stable vitals, the return of mental clarity, the ability to tolerate liquids, and comprehension of discharge instructions.

Complications

The most common complication during procedural sedation is respiratory depression. Continuous monitoring of oxygen levels and respiratory effort is essential for early detection of airway problems. If necessary, the physician should intervene by managing the airway and administering bag-valve-mask ventilation. End-tidal $CO_2$ monitoring is a valuable tool to identify hypoventilation before hypoxia becomes evident on pulse oximetry.

Other possible complications include nausea and vomiting, which can lead to aspiration. To prevent this, the patient's airway should be protected, and suctioning may be required. Inadequate sedation (failure to achieve sufficient analgesia or amnesia) can make the procedure more difficult, while prolonged sedation may occur if repeated doses of sedative agents are administered. Careful titration of medications, with regular monitoring, can minimize these risks.

Common Medications Used in Procedural Sedation:

1. Midazolam (Benzodiazepine): Administered at a dose of 0.02-0.1 mg/kg intravenously, midazolam provides sedation, amnesia, and anxiolysis. Its effects start within 2 minutes and last for about 20-30 minutes. Side effects can

include apnea and hypotension, but these can be reversed with flumazenil, a benzodiazepine antagonist.

2. Morphine (Opioid): Given at 0.1-0.2 mg/kg intravenously, morphine primarily provides analgesia. It begins working within 2 minutes and lasts for 3-4 hours. It can cause histamine release, leading to potential allergic reactions or hypotension. Naloxone is the reversal agent for morphine overdose.

3. Fentanyl (Opioid): At a dose of 0.5-1 μg/kg up to a total dose of 2-3 μg/kg intravenously, fentanyl provides analgesia and mild sedation. The effects are rapid, beginning in 2 minutes, and last about 30 minutes. Common side effects include respiratory depression and chest rigidity, which can be reversed with naloxone.

4. Ketamine (PCP Derivative): Administered at 0.5-1 mg/kg intravenously or 3-5 mg/kg intramuscularly, ketamine offers sedation, amnesia, analgesia, and anxiolysis. Its onset is very fast, occurring within 1 minute, with effects lasting 1-2 hours. Side effects include increased secretions, tachycardia, and potential emergence reactions. Ketamine has no specific reversal agent.

5. Etomidate (Imidazole Derivative): Given at a dose of 0.1-0.2 mg/kg intravenously, etomidate provides sedation, amnesia, and anxiolysis. Its effects begin within 30 seconds and last for 10-30 minutes. Myoclonus (muscle jerks) and apnea are possible side effects, but there is no specific reversal agent.

6. Propofol (Phenol Compound): Administered at 1-2 mg/kg intravenously, propofol provides sedation and amnesia, with effects starting in 40 seconds and lasting for 3-5 minutes. It can cause

hypotension, bradycardia, and pain at the injection site. Propofol has no reversal agent.

In addition, there is a highlights two reversal agents:

Flumazenil: Used to reverse benzodiazepine effects, flumazenil can be administered at 0.2 mg intravenously, which may be repeated up to 1 mg. Its onset is 1-2 minutes, and its effects last for about 45 minutes. However, it may cause seizures or withdrawal symptoms in chronic benzodiazepine users.

Naloxone: A reversal agent for opioid effects, naloxone can be administered in doses of 0.1-2 mg intravenously. It works within minutes to reverse opioid-induced respiratory depression and sedation.

Suggested Readings:

1. American College of Emergency Physicians. Clinical policy for procedural sedation and analgesia in the emergency department. Ann Emerg Med. 1998;31:663-677.

2. Deitch K, et al. Does end-tidal $CO_2$ monitoring during emergency department procedural sedation and analgesia with propofol decrease the incidence of hypoxic events? Ann Emerg Med. 2010;55:258-264.

3. Green SM, et al. Fasting and emergency department procedural sedation and analgesia: a consensus-based clinical practice advisory. Ann Emerg Med. 2007;49:454-461.

## Chapter 5
## Lumbar Puncture

A lumbar puncture (LP) is a clinical procedure performed primarily to diagnose central nervous system (CNS) infections, such as meningitis, or to investigate conditions like subarachnoid hemorrhage (SAH). This technique can also relieve cerebrospinal fluid (CSF) pressure, help diagnose idiopathic intracranial hypertension, and assist in evaluating demyelinating diseases, inflammatory CNS conditions, or metastatic cancer affecting the CNS.

Key Requirements and Contraindications

Proper execution of an LP depends on precise knowledge of anatomical landmarks and maintaining sterile technique. Key contraindications to LP include infections at the intended puncture site and any intracranial mass that could increase intracranial pressure. A non-contrast head CT is essential to rule out an intracranial mass in patients presenting with altered mental states, focal neurological signs, signs of increased ICP (such as papilledema), recent seizure, age over 60, or those who are immunocompromised. Conditions like bleeding disorders are relative contraindications, requiring careful evaluation and sometimes correction of coagulation status before the procedure.

Procedure and Technique

Typically, an LP kit includes a spinal needle, smaller needles for anesthetic administration, collection tubes, and other necessary supplies. The needle is inserted into the lumbar interspace at a slight upward angle, advancing through three key ligaments until the subarachnoid space is reached. Correct positioning and careful needle manipulation help minimize complications, and the needle's bevel orientation can reduce the risk of persistent CSF leakage, which is associated with post-LP headache.

Upon reaching the subarachnoid space, a manometer may be used to measure CSF pressure, which normally ranges from 7-18 cm $H_2O$. CSF is collected in multiple tubes for various diagnostic tests, including cell counts, glucose, and protein levels, as well as for bacterial culture and Gram staining. When anatomical challenges are present, such as obesity or joint degeneration, imaging guidance like fluoroscopy or ultrasound may facilitate accurate needle placement.

Potential Complications

Complications of an LP can include trauma to the dura or arachnoid vessels, sometimes causing a "traumatic tap" with red blood cells in the CSF. A comparison of red blood cell count from the first to last CSF tube can help differentiate a traumatic tap from a true SAH, where xanthochromia is present. Rare but serious risks include spinal hematomas, particularly in patients with coagulation disorders, and brain herniation in cases of undiagnosed intracranial mass.

Post-LP headache is the most common complication, affecting 20-70% of patients, particularly younger adults. These headaches, often positional, can persist for days and may require treatment, such as an epidural blood patch, if prolonged. Other potential issues include mild back pain from needle insertion trauma and, less commonly, infections due to contamination or improper sterile technique, leading to cellulitis or abscess formation.

Summary

A lumbar puncture is a valuable diagnostic and therapeutic procedure with a well-established protocol for safe execution. Adhering to contraindications and employing sterile techniques minimize risks, making it an effective tool in CNS assessment and management.

# Chapter 6
# Laceration Repair

Key Insights:

Optimal wound closure timing should balance infection risk against potential scarring.

Prioritize foreign body removal before wound closure.

## Indications

Consider closure for any wound deeper than a superficial abrasion to enhance cosmetic results, preserve viable tissue, and improve tensile strength. Closure methods include sutures, tissue adhesive, or staples:

Tissue adhesive works well for low-tension, hemostatic wounds with a minimal infection risk.

Staples suit relatively straight lacerations on the extremities, trunk, or scalp.

Contraindications

The decision to repair a laceration depends on various factors involving the patient's health and the wound itself:

Patient-related factors: Age (higher infection rates and slower healing in the elderly), malnutrition, and immunosuppression (e.g., diabetes).

Wound-related factors: Timing, location, type of injury, and contamination level. Bacterial counts increase 3-6 hours post-injury; ideally, wounds should be closed promptly. However, there is no definitive evidence-based timeframe for closure.

Facial and scalp wounds, with their excellent blood supply, can safely be closed up to 24 hours after injury. Infection rates are higher in the upper (4%) and lower extremities (7%), where a 6-12-hour closure window is common.

Additional considerations

Blunt or crushing injuries involve more tissue damage and carry higher infection risk than sharp injuries.

Puncture wounds and bite wounds (e.g., dog, cat, human bites) have elevated infection risks due to embedded bacteria. Bite wounds generally aren't closed unless in cosmetically sensitive areas, like the face.

Staples and tissue adhesive are unsuitable for deep wounds needing layered closure or for use on mucosal areas, the scalp, or over joints without immobilization.

Equipment

Essential supplies for wound closure include:

Povidone-iodine solution

Local anesthetic (1% lidocaine, with or without epinephrine)

A 25- or 27-gauge needle and syringe

Irrigation tools, including a 60-mL syringe and an irrigation shield or 18-gauge angiocatheter (although tap water may suffice for simple wounds in some cases).

Instruments needed are a needle driver, tissue forceps, and scissors. Use the smallest suitable monofilament suture to minimize scarring, usually 4-0 for the torso and extremities and 6-0 for facial wounds.

Procedure

1. Timing: Wound healing methods include:

Primary intention: Standard repair where wound edges are immediately closed with sutures, staples, or adhesive.

Secondary intention: Wounds are left open to heal naturally if infection risk is high.

Tertiary intention (delayed primary closure): For contaminated wounds, the wound is cleaned, then sutured after a few days to reduce infection risk.

2. Wound Preparation: Adequate lighting and hemostasis are necessary. Conduct a thorough neurovascular exam before administering anesthesia, assess tendon function if relevant, and explore for foreign bodies or deeper injuries. Suspected foreign materials (e.g., glass) may require radiography, with additional imaging

needed for non-radiopaque objects like plastic or wood.

For wounds in hair-covered areas, clip hair rather than shave, or apply antibacterial ointment to part hair, aiding visualization and reducing infection risk. Avoid hair removal from eyebrows or the hairline to prevent abnormal regrowth.

Clean wound edges with povidone-iodine, avoiding direct wound exposure to the solution as it hinders healing. Buffer lidocaine with bicarbonate to reduce injection pain (1 mL bicarbonate per 9 mL lidocaine) and apply promptly. Infiltrate lidocaine around wound edges or use a field block approach for contaminated wounds to minimize infection risk.

3. Wound Closure: Principles for simple interrupted sutures include:

Insert the needle perpendicularly to encourage wound edge eversion, which supports faster healing and reduces depressed scarring.

Avoid excessive tension to prevent ischemia at wound edges, indicated by blanching. Begin in the wound's center, working outward, ensuring uniform stitch spacing and depth.

Vertical and horizontal mattress sutures provide excellent edge approximation and wound eversion for tensioned or challenging areas, like joints or hands. Vertical sutures are also useful for scalp bleeding but may constrict tissues if overly tight.

Deep sutures are essential for wounds with multiple tissue layers or large gaping wounds. They reduce superficial skin tension and use absorbable suture material. Only apply the minimal number of deep sutures to close the wound edges and minimize infection risk.

Staples require edge eversion before applying with consistent spacing, while tissue adhesive is applied in multiple layers on dry, cleaned wounds. Avoid adhesive contact within the wound itself.

Aftercare: A moist environment with topical antibiotics enhances epithelialization and infection prevention, though they aren't used after adhesive application. Prophylactic oral antibiotics are indicated for heavily contaminated wounds, bites, high-risk areas, or immunocompromised patients.

For tetanus prophylaxis, patients with updated vaccinations receive a booster (Td, 0.5 mL IM) only if the last dose was over ten years ago for clean wounds, or five years for more severe cases. Tetanus immune globulin is given for inadequately immunized patients with contaminated wounds.

Dress the wound with topical ointment (e.g., bacitracin) and a sterile covering for optimal healing.

Suggested Reading

1. Desai, S., Stone, S.C., & Carter, W.A. Wound Preparation. In: Tintinalli, J.E., Stapczynski, J.S., Ma, O.J., Cline, D.M., Cydulka, R.K., & Meckler, G.D. (Eds.), Tintinalli's Emergency Medicine: A Comprehensive Study Guide (7th ed., pp. 301-306). New York, NY: McGraw-Hill; 2011.

2. Singer, A.J., & Hollander, J.E. Methods for Wound Closure. In: Tintinalli, J.E., Stapczynski, J.S., Ma, O.J., Cline, D.M., Cydulka, R.K., & Meckler, G.D. (Eds.), Tintinalli's Emergency Medicine: A Comprehensive Study Guide (7th ed., pp. 306-315). New York, NY: McGraw-Hill; 2011.

3. Singer, A.J., Hollander, J.E., & Quinn, J.V. Evaluation and Management of Traumatic Lacerations. New England Journal of Medicine, 1997;337:1142-1148.

## Chapter 7

## Needle and Tube Thoracostomy: Key Guidelines and Procedure

Key Points

Avoid mistaking pulmonary blebs or bullae for pneumothorax.

The neurovascular bundle is positioned below each rib; enter the thoracic cavity above the rib to avoid injury.

Indications

Needle thoracostomy is critical for the emergency decompression of a suspected tension pneumothorax. Following this, tube thoracostomy may be warranted for simple pneumothorax, traumatic hemothorax, or large pleural effusions with respiratory compromise.

Contraindications

Pulmonary blebs or bullae, large air-filled spaces with thin walls, may appear similar to a pneumothorax on a chest X-ray. These formations, often seen in individuals with severe chronic obstructive pulmonary disease (COPD), are frequently found at the lung apex. Confirmation of pneumothorax is essential prior to thoracostomy placement to avoid complications. For scenarios where tube thoracostomy may be substituted with conservative management.

Equipment

For needle thoracostomy, a 12- to 16-gauge angiocath of 3 to 4.5 inches and a 5-10 mL syringe are required. Tube thoracostomy necessitates a larger 36- to 40-F tube for adult hemothorax, or 20- to 24-F tube for children. For simple pneumothorax, use an 18- to 28-F tube for adults or a 14- to 16-F tube for children. Additional supplies include antiseptic solution, sterile drapes, gloves, 20 mL of 1% lidocaine with epinephrine, a scalpel, clamps, needle driver, suture materials, and a suction apparatus.

Procedure

1. Needle Thoracostomy

Cleanse the upper chest skin. Insert the catheter-over-needle at the second intercostal space above the third rib at the midclavicular line. A rush of air confirms tension pneumothorax and an improvement in vitals indicates successful decompression. Follow with tube thoracostomy.

2. Tube Thoracostomy

Position the patient with the affected arm above their head. Prepare the area around the fourth intercostal space at the mid-axillary line. Administer local anesthesia with lidocaine at the skin, deeper layers, and intercostal muscles down to the parietal pleura. An incision of 2-3 cm is made, and a large curved clamp tunnels through the tissues to the pleural cavity. Insert a gloved finger to confirm absence of adhesions. Insert the chest tube, ensuring the tube's drainage holes are positioned within the thoracic cavity. Secure the tube and attach it to suction. A post-procedure chest X-ray is required to verify placement and confirm re-expansion.

Complications

Needle Thoracostomy: The most frequent issue is decompression failure. Body habitus may necessitate a longer catheter (4.5 cm) if the standard length is insufficient to reach the pleural space.

Tube Thoracostomy

Infection: High rates of infection in trauma cases (up to 25%) emphasize the need for strict sterility.

Tube Displacement: Never reposition a displaced tube; instead, insert a new one.

Bleeding: Can arise from superficial vessels or injury to the lung or abdominal organs.

Improper Tube Placement: Issues such as kinking or subcutaneous placement can hinder drainage or cause persistent air leaks.

Reexpansion Pulmonary Edema: This rare but serious complication occurs when a collapsed lung expands too rapidly. If the lung has been collapsed for an extended period, use a water seal to achieve gradual reexpansion.

Suggested Reading

1. Brunette, P.H., et al. Pulmonary Trauma. In: Tintinalli, J.E., Stapczynski, J.S., Ma, O.J., Cline, D.M., Cydulka, R.K., Meckler, G.D. (Eds.), Tintinalli's Emergency Medicine: A Comprehensive Study Guide (7th ed., pp. 1744-1758). New York, NY: McGraw-Hill; 2011.

2. Joseph, K.T. Tube Thoracostomy. In: Reichman, E.F., & Simon, R.R. (Eds.), Emergency Medicine Procedures (1st ed., pp. 226-236). New York, NY: McGraw-Hill; 2004.

# Chapter 8
# Introduction to Emergency Ultrasonography

Key Points

Emergency physicians' use of ultrasound has grown significantly over the last decades.

Key emergency uses include trauma assessment, abdominal aortic aneurysm (AAA) detection, ectopic pregnancy, gallbladder, and kidney evaluation, as well as procedural guidance (e.g., IV access).

Indications

Emergency ultrasound (EUS) is conducted bedside by emergency physicians to rapidly address focused diagnostic questions, assist in invasive procedures, and monitor treatment response. The 2008 guidelines from the

American College of Emergency Physicians outline eleven core applications of EUS. The primary uses include:

1. Abdominal and Chest Trauma: The Focused Assessment with Sonography for Trauma (FAST) scan quickly evaluates for fluid in the pericardial, pleural, and peritoneal spaces. The extended FAST scan can also detect pneumothorax.

2. Ectopic Pregnancy: EUS is effective in ruling out ectopic pregnancy when an intrauterine pregnancy is identified, addressing symptoms like first-trimester abdominal/pelvic pain or vaginal bleeding.

3. Abdominal Aortic Aneurysm (AAA): EUS helps rule out AAA in patients with vague abdominal or back pain, reducing the need for CT scans. For patients with hypotension and abdominal pain, EUS can expedite the AAA

diagnosis and facilitate prompt surgical intervention.

4. Acute Cholecystitis: Physical examination and lab results for acute cholecystitis are often inconclusive; however, EUS can confirm or exclude the diagnosis, leading to faster clinical decisions.

5. Renal Colic: In cases of flank pain with hematuria, EUS can identify hydronephrosis, supporting a diagnosis of nephrolithiasis without additional imaging.

6. Procedural Guidance: EUS assists in performing various procedures, including central and peripheral line placement, lumbar puncture, abscess drainage, and guided pericardiocentesis, thoracentesis, and paracentesis.

Contraindications

EUS use may be limited by factors such as patient obesity, excessive bowel gas, or limited physician experience. In cases where EUS does not answer the clinical question or unexpected findings arise, further testing may be required. EUS is a valuable tool but is not a substitute for more comprehensive imaging when needed.

Equipment

EUS functions similarly to sonar technology: sound waves are emitted, travel through tissues, reflect off structures, and return to the probe. These echoes are then processed to create a visual image.

Frequency: Higher frequency probes (8-10 MHz) provide detailed images of superficial structures (e.g., for line placements), while lower frequency probes (2-5 MHz) are better suited for deep thoracic and abdominal scans.

Echogenicity: Image quality is based on how well different tissues reflect sound waves. Dense structures, like bone, appear bright, while fluid-filled areas (such as blood) appear dark.

Orientation: EUS requires careful attention to probe positioning. In longitudinal (sagittal) orientation, the probe marker points to the head, showing the head on the screen's left and feet on the right. In transverse (coronal) views, the probe points right, displaying images similar to CT scans.

Ultrasound Modes

Brightness (B) mode is the most widely used, while Motion (M) mode captures movement, such as a fetal heartbeat. Doppler and color flow modes assess blood flow.

Procedure

A basic FAST examination involves scanning the abdomen and lower thorax while the patient lies supine, and the physician operates from the patient's right. Specific views include:

1. Subxiphoid View: The probe is placed below the sternum, aiming leftward, to identify pericardial fluid.

2. Right Upper Quadrant (RUQ) View: The probe is placed at the mid-axillary line to assess the right hemithorax and hepatorenal (Morison's) pouch.

3. Left Upper Quadrant (LUQ) View: Positioned along the posterior axillary line, this view assesses the left hemithorax, subphrenic, and splenorenal spaces.

4. Pelvic View: With the probe above the pubic symphysis, this view examines the rectouterine

pouch in females or the retrovesicular space in males.

Complications

Complications with EUS typically result from poor image clarity or misinterpretation rather than the ultrasound procedure itself.

Suggested Reading

1. American College of Emergency Physicians. "Emergency Ultrasound Guidelines." Ann Emerg Med, 2009.

2. Hoffmann, R., et al. "Management of Sonography in Blunt Abdominal Trauma." Unfallchirurg, 1989.

3. Ma, O.J., et al. "Prospective Analysis of a Rapid Trauma Ultrasound Examination

Performed by Emergency Physicians." J Trauma, 1995.

4. Melniker, L.A., et al. "Randomized Controlled Clinical Trial of Point-of-Care, Limited Ultrasonography for Trauma in the Emergency Department." Ann Emerg Med, 2006.

## Chapter 9
## Emergency Medical Services

Key Takeaways:

Emergency Medical Services (EMS) extend medical care beyond traditional healthcare facilities, into the prehospital environment.

The U.S. EMS Systems Act of 1973 was pivotal in establishing essential elements that must be met for EMS funding.

Introduction:

Emergency Medical Services (EMS) is a specialized area of healthcare dedicated to providing medical care outside hospital settings. EMS can refer specifically to prehospital care or encompass an entire integrated system, including hospitals as primary care providers. The U.S.

EMS Systems Act of 1973 introduced 15 foundational elements required for EMS systems to receive federal support, shaping the structure of EMS programs.

Workforce:

EMS workforce composition is influenced by population density. Urban areas generally have paid EMS personnel who may work within government agencies or as public safety officers in large public venues (e.g., airports, amusement parks). In contrast, suburban, rural, and wilderness areas more commonly rely on volunteer EMS providers.

Training:

The U.S. Department of Transportation's National Highway Traffic Safety Administration (NHTSA) provides a standardized curriculum for EMS providers, which defines four certification levels:

1. Emergency Medical Responder (EMR): First responders trained to deliver basic life-saving care, including CPR, hemorrhage control, and AED use.

2. Emergency Medical Technician (EMT): EMTs provide patient transport and additional care, such as administering certain medications.

3. Advanced EMT (AEMT): Under physician direction, AEMTs can perform intravenous access, electrocardiogram (ECG) interpretation, and administer a broader range of medications.

4. Paramedic: Paramedics perform advanced medical procedures and administer a wider variety of drugs, including those needed for pain management and critical conditions.

Communications and Access to Care:

The "911" emergency number, established in the 1970s, serves as a universal access point for emergency care. Trained dispatchers gather essential details to prioritize and allocate resources for a response and may also provide pre-arrival instructions, such as guiding a caller in performing CPR.

Transportation

EMS transport vehicles are equipped to align with the intended response and provider's training scope. Basic Life Support (BLS) units carry essential supplies for basic care, while Advanced Life Support (ALS) units support paramedics with advanced equipment. Specialized transport units, such as those equipped for critical care, can handle patients needing continuous IV infusions or ventilators. Air transport options include helicopters and fixed-wing aircraft, suitable for situations where timely ground transport is impractical or where specialized care is needed.

Critical Care Facilities

Prehospital patients are typically transported to the nearest appropriate facility, but factors like hospital overcrowding or availability of specialized services (e.g., trauma, cardiac, or stroke centers) may affect destination choice. Designated facilities with specialty care for time-sensitive conditions, such as trauma or burns, are prioritized.

Public Safety Coordination

EMS operations are often collaborative efforts involving police, fire, and EMS personnel. EMS structures may vary, including fire-based, third-service, private, or hospital-based EMS providers, each with unique roles and capabilities.

Community Involvement

EMS frequently engages in public education, such as CPR training and safety awareness, and community members often contribute to EMS decision-making, highlighting EMS's role as both a public health and safety resource.

Patient Transfer and Documentation

EMS's primary role is to ensure timely patient transfer to appropriate medical facilities. The Emergency Medical Treatment and Active Labor Act (EMTALA) mandates stabilization before inter-facility transfer, with hospitals needing to approve transfers. Despite the growing use of electronic medical records, variability in data collection and documentation remains a barrier to EMS research and patient outcome tracking.

Quality Control and Disaster Preparedness

EMS protocols undergo regular updates based on scientific advances and changing community needs. Continuous quality improvement processes help identify areas for improvement.

For large-scale incidents, protocols like "Simple Triage and Rapid Treatment" (START) aid in assessing injury severity and prioritizing care.

Mutual Aid

Neighboring EMS systems often have mutual aid agreements, enabling coordinated responses during large-scale emergencies. Effective interagency communication and compatible equipment are vital to these partnerships.

Suggested Readings:

1. Emergency Medical Services: Clinical Practice and Systems Oversight by the National Association of EMS Physicians

2. Tintinalli's Emergency Medicine: A Comprehensive Study Guide (7th edition), which includes an EMS-focused section by Mechem et al.

3. The National EMS Scope of Practice Model, published by the National Highway Traffic Safety Administration

# Chapter 10
# Cardiopulmonary Arrest

Key Insights:

Cardiac disease stands as the leading non-traumatic death cause in the U.S.

Annually, over 300,000 cases of sudden cardiac death (SCD) occur in the U.S., with survival rates influenced by timely intervention and underlying factors.

Introduction

Cardiopulmonary arrest is characterized by loss of consciousness, apnea, and absence of a pulse. Sudden cardiac death (SCD) is often linked to coronary artery disease (CAD), although only 20-40% of cardiac arrests involve acute thrombosis. Around 25% of arrests are due to non-cardiac causes (e.g., pulmonary embolism, respiratory arrest, drowning, overdose). Initial rhythm is frequently ventricular fibrillation (VF), followed by asystole and pulseless electrical activity (PEA). Patients with CAD risk factors face a fourfold increase in SCD risk, while those with known heart disease have a six- to tenfold increase. Structural heart diseases like cardiomyopathy or myocarditis contribute to about 10% of SCD cases, while another 10% occur in patients without CAD or structural heart disease, attributed to conditions like Brugada syndrome, prolonged QT syndrome, and inherited ventricular tachycardia.

Key risk factors for SCD include smoking, diabetes, hypertension, dyslipidemia, and family history. Moderate alcohol use may be protective, whereas heavy drinking is a risk factor. Despite advancements in resuscitation, the survival rate for out-of-hospital SCD is low (3-8%), with survival highly dependent on the initial cardiac rhythm. Patients presenting with VF have a significantly higher discharge survival rate (34%) than those with asystole (0-2%).

## Clinical Evaluation and Diagnostic Approach

### 1. History

Gather history from available sources like paramedics or family, focusing on medications, medical history, allergies, and events preceding the arrest.

### 2. Physical Examination

Continuation of chest compressions and ventilation is critical during examination. If intubated, confirm tube position using end-tidal $CO_2$.

### 3. Diagnostic Studies

Laboratory Tests: If spontaneous circulation returns (ROSC), evaluate with a complete blood count, electrolytes, renal function, troponin, coagulation studies, arterial blood gas, and lactate.

Imaging: Post-ROSC, perform a chest x-ray to assess tube placement and an ECG to check for ischemia.

4. Procedures

Pericardiocentesis: Indicated for suspected cardiac tamponade in PEA. Ultrasound guidance is helpful. Insert a spinal needle subxiphoid, aiming toward the left shoulder, and aspirate blood.

Needle Thoracostomy: For suspected tension pneumothorax in PEA, insert an 18-gauge needle into the second intercostal space at the midclavicular line, followed by a tube thoracostomy upon ROSC.

Management and Treatment

1. Defibrillation

For VF or pulseless VT, defibrillation is critical. Success rates are over 90% if conducted within one minute of onset but decrease by 10% for each minute delayed.

2. Chest Compressions

Continuous, high-quality chest compressions (depth 1.5-2 inches at a rate >100/min) are essential. Interruptions should be minimized, with brief rhythm checks every 2 minutes and compression during defibrillator charging.

3. Airway Management

Airway obstruction from the tongue is common in unconscious patients. Use a jaw thrust or chin lift, followed by bag-valve-mask ventilation until advanced airway tools are ready. Intubation should be quick to avoid interrupting compressions.

4. Pharmacologic Intervention

Vasopressors: Administer 1 mg epinephrine IV every 3-5 minutes. If no IV access is available, deliver epinephrine through the endotracheal tube at 2-2.5 times the IV dose.

Antidysrhythmics: Amiodarone, initially 300 mg IV push followed by 150 mg if needed, is effective in refractory VT/VF. For torsades de pointes, administer magnesium sulfate, 2 g IV.

5. Post-Resuscitation Care

Patients with ROSC who remain comatose should receive therapeutic hypothermia (33°C for 24 hours, with gradual rewarming).

Disposition

Admit all ROSC patients to the ICU or cardiac care unit for post-resuscitation management and evaluation of underlying causes. If CAD or acute coronary syndrome is suspected as the cause, interventions such as percutaneous coronary intervention should be considered.

Suggested Readings:

1. 67sField JM, Hazinski MF, Sayre MR, et al. "Executive Summary: 2010 American Heart Association Guidelines for Cardiopulmonary Resuscitation and Emergency Cardiovascular Care," Circulation, 2010; 122:S640-S656.

2. Neumar RW, Otto CW, Link MS, et al. "Adult Advanced Cardiovascular Life Support: 2010 American Heart

Association Guidelines," Circulation, 2010;122:S729-S767.

3. Zomato, JP. "Sudden Cardiac Death," in Tintinalli's Emergency Medicine: A Comprehensive Study Guide, 7th ed., McGraw-Hill, 2011, pp. 63-67.

## Chapter 11
## Airway Management - Key Insights and Evidence-Based Practice

Key Points

Rapid Sequence Intubation (RSI): RSI remains the most widely recommended method for intubation in emergency settings due to its efficiency.

Clinical Decision-Making: Deciding when to intubate should rely on clinical assessment, supplemented by predictive factors for airway difficulty when possible.

Introduction

Effective airway management is essential and relies on recognizing compromised airways early, identifying potential barriers to effective ventilation, and using appropriate techniques to ensure airway security. The decision to proceed with intubation is based on three primary indicators: (1) inability to protect the airway from aspiration or obstruction, (2) failure to oxygenate blood (hypoxemia), and (3) inability to eliminate carbon dioxide (hypercapnia). Other considerations for intubation include reducing respiratory effort (e.g., in sepsis), controlling intracranial pressure, or managing patients requiring diagnostic imaging but who cannot cooperate due to altered mental status.

Airway management techniques range from simple positional adjustments to surgical interventions. Basic life support measures such as the head-tilt or chin-lift maneuvers can often relieve obstruction, while oropharyngeal or nasopharyngeal adjuncts serve as practical, although sometimes underused, aids in securing the airway. When these methods are ineffective, endotracheal intubation is necessary. RSI, combining pre-intubation treatment with induction and paralysis, is particularly favored in emergency departments.

## Clinical Approach to Airway Management

### Criteria for Intubation

Key indications for endotracheal intubation include:

1. Airway Protection: To prevent aspiration.

2. Oxygenation and Ventilation Failure: Due to hypoxemia or hypercapnia.

3. Alternative Measures: Consider techniques like cricothyrotomy if initial intubation efforts fail and ventilation remains inadequate.

### Techniques and Equipment Selection

The initial approach involves bag-valve-mask (BVM) ventilation, which requires an unobstructed airway and a secure mask seal. Techniques such as the head-tilt chin-lift or jaw-thrust (in trauma cases) are essential, along with airway adjuncts if necessary. RSI follows a preoxygenation phase to mitigate aspiration risks, followed by preparation of equipment, including choosing an appropriate endotracheal tube (ETT) size.

Common Equipment: Laryngoscopes, various blade types (Macintosh for indirect epiglottis manipulation or Miller for direct epiglottis lifting), and ETT sizes tailored for adults and children. Generally, cuffed ETTs are preferred, although size may vary depending on age and anatomy.

Clinical Presentation

History

In emergencies, immediate airway assessment takes precedence over history. When possible, determine risk factors that may complicate BVM or ETT placement. Factors that complicate BVM include facial trauma, obesity, or asthma. ETT placement can be hindered by conditions like limited neck mobility (e.g., due to rheumatoid arthritis), structural deformities from head or neck tumors, or tissue swelling (e.g., angioedema).

Physical Examination

A rapid airway evaluation is critical for all unstable patients, particularly in trauma cases where cervical spine injury must be assumed until proven otherwise. Key examination points include assessing for facial trauma or anatomical barriers like a beard, examining the oropharynx for obstructive factors (e.g., dentures, overbite), and applying the "3-3-2" rule to anticipate difficulty in ETT placement. This rule assesses mouth opening, chin-to-neck distance, and mandible-to-thyroid distance, with any limitations suggesting intubation challenges.

Diagnostic Studies

Blood gas analysis (for hypercapnia) and pulse oximetry (for hypoxemia) provide insight into respiratory function. However, normal values in deteriorating patients should not delay intubation. In addition, post-intubation chest x-rays verify ETT placement, aiming for a location approximately 2 cm above the carina to avoid the right bronchus.

Medical Decision-Making

Identify reversible causes of airway compromise, such as hypoglycemia or opioid overdose, that can sometimes rapidly restore consciousness and airway control. Recognize patients likely to present a difficult airway and adapt intubation approaches accordingly.

Procedures

Bag-Valve-Mask Ventilation

Effective BVM ventilation requires an open airway and a tight mask seal. The use of high-flow oxygen can achieve approximately 90% FiO2. Techniques should adapt to trauma cases to avoid worsening injuries, such as using a jaw-thrust instead of a head-tilt.

Rapid Sequence Intubation

Preoxygenate patients using a non-rebreather mask to reduce stomach insufflation and aspiration risk. Prepare all necessary equipment, select an ETT size appropriate for patient age and condition, and ensure the laryngoscope light functions. RSI medications fall into pretreatment agents (e.g., lidocaine for head injury patients), induction agents (e.g., etomidate), and paralytics (e.g., succinylcholine), each tailored to achieve quick sedation and paralysis.

In specific cases, modifications to RSI protocols may be necessary, such as pretreatment with lidocaine to mitigate ICP spikes in head injury patients, using atropine for children to avoid bradycardia, or using opioids for patients where blood pressure surges are dangerous. Although certain pretreatment regimens have been controversial, evidence supports their tailored use in high-risk situations.

Suggested Readings:

1. Hedayati, T., Ross, C., & Nasr, N. (2012). Airway Procedures: Rapid Sequence Intubation. Simon, R.R., Ross, C.R., Bowman, S.H., & Wakim, P.E. (Eds.), Cook County Manual of Emergency Procedures (1st ed., pp. 14–21). Philadelphia, PA: Lippincott Williams & Wilkins.

2. Roman, A.M. (2011). Noninvasive Airway Management. In Tintinalli, J.E., Stapczynski, J.S., Ma, O.J., Clince, D.M., Cydulka, R.K., & Meckler, G.D. (Eds.), Tintinalli's Emergency Medicine: A

Comprehensive Study Guide (7th ed., pp. 183–190). New York, NY: McGraw-Hill.


3. Vissers, R.J., & Danzl, D.F. (2011). Tracheal Intubation and Mechanical Ventilation. In Tintinalli, J.E., Stapczynski, J.S., Ma, O.J., Clince, D.M., Cydulka, R.K., & Meckler, G.D. (Eds.), Tintinalli's Emergency Medicine: A Comprehensive Study Guide (7th ed., pp. 198–215). New York, NY: McGraw-Hill.

## Chapter 12
## Shock Management in Clinical Practice

Key Insights

Do not delay diagnosing shock until hypotension is evident.

Prompt identification and aggressive treatment initiation are critical to improving survival rates.

Introduction

Each year, over a million patients in U.S. emergency rooms experience shock. Despite advancements in critical care, mortality remains high. Shock arises when the circulatory system fails to supply sufficient oxygen and nutrients to meet the body's metabolic demands. Initially reversible, prolonged low blood flow can lead to cellular hypoxia and biochemical imbalance. Shock is clinically categorized as follows:

hypovolemic, cardiogenic, obstructive, and distributive.

Hypovolemic Shock: Caused by a decrease in blood volume, due to severe dehydration or hemorrhage. This form is most prevalent among patients under 40.

Cardiogenic Shock: Results from heart failure, often due to a major myocardial infarction impairing at least 40% of the heart muscle.

Obstructive Shock: Stems from an extracardiac obstruction (e.g., pericardial tamponade, tension pneumothorax, pulmonary embolism) that restricts venous return.

Distributive Shock: Occurs from uncontrolled vascular tone loss, as seen in sepsis, anaphylaxis, or neurogenic shock.

Neurogenic shock, often linked to cervical spine injuries, manifests as hypotension and paradoxical bradycardia and should be diagnosed by excluding other causes. Elderly, immunocompromised, and high-risk patients may show only vague symptoms, yet require swift intervention due to high mortality rates (30-90%).

Pathophysiology

Shock progression follows three primary phases:

1. Autonomic Response: The body raises cardiac output, redirecting blood to vital organs (brain, heart) while minimizing flow to less critical areas (e.g., skin, kidneys).

2. Cellular Hypoxia: Persistent low oxygen forces cells to shift from aerobic to less efficient anaerobic metabolism, leading to acidosis from lactate accumulation.

3. Inflammatory Cascade: Injured cells release inflammatory mediators, leading to systemic inflammatory response syndrome (SIRS) marked by fever, tachycardia, rapid breathing, and elevated white cell count.

## Clinical Presentation

### History

Symptoms may be nonspecific, such as fatigue and confusion. A thorough history—including medication, immune status, and cardiovascular health—helps assess risks and possible triggers.

### Physical Examination

Key signs include hypotension and tachycardia, though compensatory mechanisms may mask these early on. Changes in mental status, jugular vein distention, heart murmurs, lung sounds, and skin temperature can help distinguish shock types. For example:

Distributive Shock: Warm, flushed skin.

Other Types (e.g., hypovolemic): Cool, mottled extremities.

Diagnostic Workup

Laboratory Tests: No single test diagnoses shock. Key indicators include:

White Blood Cell Count: Bands >10% indicate infection.

Lactate Levels: High levels (>4 mmol/L) suggest hypoxia and predict mortality, especially in septic shock.

Other relevant tests include cardiac markers, coagulation profiles, and toxicology screens. Cultures (e.g., blood, urine) should be obtained when sepsis is suspected.

Imaging: While no imaging is definitive, certain findings aid diagnosis:

Chest X-ray: May show infiltrates (sepsis), an enlarged cardiac silhouette (tamponade), or signs of pneumothorax.

Bedside Ultrasound: Useful for identifying abdominal trauma, pregnancy complications, aortic aneurysm, or tamponade.

CT Scans: Often preferred for diagnosing pulmonary embolism, aortic dissection, or abdominal pathology.

Procedures and Medical Decision Making

Intubation may be necessary to lower respiratory effort and metabolic demands. Central lines enable rapid fluid, vasopressor administration, and central venous pressure monitoring. Rapid diagnosis of shock type and cause is essential, with management focusing on restoring circulation and addressing the underlying issue.

Treatment Strategies

The goal is twofold: stabilize cellular function and resolve the cause of shock. General measures include supplemental oxygen and IV access for fluid resuscitation. Specific treatments vary by shock type:

Hypovolemic Shock

Restore blood volume promptly with normal saline and, if needed, packed red blood cells. Caution with fluid in trauma patients to avoid rebleeding.

Distributive Shock

Septic Shock: Administer fluids to achieve a central venous pressure (CVP) of 8-12 mmHg, and add vasopressors like norepinephrine to maintain a mean arterial pressure (MAP) >65 mmHg. Initiate broad-spectrum antibiotics and perform surgical intervention as needed.

Neurogenic Shock: After ruling out other causes, expand blood volume with saline boluses. Dopamine may be used for vasopressor support; atropine may treat bradycardia.

Anaphylactic Shock: Immediate action with epinephrine, antihistamines, and corticosteroids, ensuring removal of any allergen.

Obstructive Shock

Cardiac Tamponade: Administer fluids followed by pericardiocentesis.

Pulmonary Embolism: Small saline boluses, followed by fibrinolysis if indicated.

Tension Pneumothorax: Emergent needle decompression is life-saving.

## Conclusion

Shock demands rapid recognition, immediate stabilization of ABCs (airway, breathing, circulation), and aggressive treatment tailored to the underlying cause. Each subtype requires specific interventions to ensure the best possible outcomes for patients in this critical state.

## Suggested Reading

1. Cherkas, D. (2011). Traumatic hemorrhagic shock: Advances in fluid management. Emergency Medicine Practice, 13(1), 1-20.

2. Dellinger, R. P., Levy, M. M., et al. (2008). Surviving Sepsis Campaign: International guidelines for the management of severe sepsis and septic shock. Critical Care Medicine, 36(8), 296-327.

3. Otero, R. M., Nguyen, H. B., & Rivers, E. P. (2011). Approach to the patient in shock. In J. E. Tintinalli, J. S. Stapczynski, D. M. Cline, O. J. Ma, R. K. Cydulka, & G. D. Meckler (Eds.), Tintinalli's Emergency Medicine: A Comprehensive Study Guide (7th ed., pp. xx-xx). New York, NY: McGraw-Hill.

4. Reynolds, H. R., & Hochman, J. S. (2008). Cardiogenic shock: Current concepts and improving outcomes. Circulation, 117(5), 686-697.

## Chapter 13
## Chest Pain Evaluation and Management

Key Points

Chest pain is a frequent reason for emergency department (ED) visits.

Rapid assessment, including an electrocardiogram (ECG) and chest X-ray, is essential for distinguishing between various critical causes of chest pain.

The primary diagnostic concern is to rule out life-threatening conditions.

Introduction

Chest pain is one of the most prevalent reasons for patient visits to the emergency department (ED). Several potentially life-threatening conditions present with chest pain, making it crucial to quickly differentiate between urgent and non-urgent causes. A systematic approach, including a comprehensive history, physical examination, and diagnostic testing, is essential for accurate diagnosis.

Pain arises from either somatic or visceral nerve fibers, with distinct characteristics for each. Somatic pain, which typically presents as sharp and localized, is often caused by conditions like pulmonary embolism, pneumothorax, musculoskeletal injury, herpes zoster, pneumonia, or pleurisy. On the other hand, visceral pain is vague, poorly localized, and may radiate to nearby structures. Conditions like acute coronary syndrome (ACS), aortic dissection, gastroesophageal reflux, and pericarditis are common causes of visceral pain.

Clinical Presentation

History

A thorough history is vital for assessing chest pain. No single symptom can definitively determine the cause of chest pain, so a detailed exploration of the pain's nature, location, and associated factors is required.

Pain Character: Sharp, stabbing pain is more typical of pulmonary embolism than ACS. Conversely, dull, pressure-like discomfort is more suggestive of ACS.

Pain Location and Radiation: Ischemic chest pain is usually located beneath the sternum or on the left side and may radiate to the left arm or jaw. A "tearing" pain radiating through the back is often seen in aortic dissection.

Pain Duration and Severity: Mild pain lasting only seconds is typically benign, while persistent pain lasting over 10 minutes is more concerning. Recurrent pain that lasts hours or days is unlikely to be cardiac in origin.

Exacerbating and Relieving Factors: Chest pain worsened by exertion and relieved by rest is suggestive of cardiac causes. Pain aggravated by deep inspiration or coughing could indicate pleurisy, a musculoskeletal issue, or pulmonary embolism. Epigastric pain worsened by meals may suggest a gastrointestinal origin, while stress-related pain could be linked to psychiatric issues.

Associated Symptoms: Nausea and sweating increase the likelihood of ACS. Other important factors to assess include a history of hypercoagulable states (suggesting pulmonary embolism) or connective tissue disorders (suggesting aortic dissection).

Physical Examination

The general appearance of the patient can provide clues. Patients with ACS or other serious conditions often appear anxious, pale, and diaphoretic. A focused physical exam should assess vital signs, the heart, lungs, abdomen, extremities, and neurologic systems.

ACS: Symptoms may include abnormal heart sounds, such as S3 or S4, and signs of pulmonary edema (e.g., rales).

Tension Pneumothorax: Look for decreased breath sounds, tracheal deviation, and respiratory distress.

Pericardial Tamponade: Look for hypotension, muffled heart sounds, jugular venous distension, and .

Pulmonary Embolism (PE): Patients may have pleuritic chest pain, dyspnea, and signs of right heart strain. Look for unilateral leg swelling indicative of deep vein thrombosis (DVT).

Aortic Dissection: Aortic dissection presents with severe, sharp pain, often radiating through the chest and back, and may be associated with a pulse deficit or a significant blood pressure difference between arms.

Diagnostic Studies

1. ECG: All patients with chest pain or symptoms suggestive of ACS should receive an ECG within 10 minutes of presentation.

2. Cardiac Markers: Troponin assays, along with CK-MB analysis, are essential for ACS diagnosis.

3. Chest X-ray: This should be obtained for most patients with chest pain. It can identify conditions like pneumothorax, pneumonia, and aortic dissection.

4. CT Angiography: This is the preferred imaging modality for diagnosing pulmonary embolism and aortic dissection. It is also useful for coronary artery disease evaluation.

5. Echocardiography: Transthoracic or transesophageal echocardiography can help assess pericardial effusions, ACS-related hypokinesis, and right ventricular strain in PE.

Medical Decision Making

A combination of history, physical examination, ECG, and chest radiography often provides enough information to exclude urgent conditions. When more data is needed, laboratory tests and an understanding of pre-test probabilities guide further decision-making.

Treatment

Acute Coronary Syndrome (ACS): Administer supplemental oxygen, aspirin (162–365 mg), and sublingual nitroglycerin (0.4 mg every 5 minutes). Early revascularization is critical, especially for patients with ST-elevation myocardial infarction (STEMI).

Aortic Dissection: Rapid heart rate and blood pressure reduction are essential. Medications aim to maintain a heart rate below 60 bpm and systolic BP under 100 mmHg, often using dual therapy to control both parameters.

Pulmonary Embolism (PE): Treatment varies based on hemodynamic stability. Stable patients should be anticoagulated with heparin, while unstable patients may require thrombolytic therapy.

Boerhaave Syndrome (Esophageal Rupture): Broad-spectrum antibiotics should be administered, followed by surgical repair.

Pneumothorax: All patients should receive supplemental oxygen. Tension pneumothorax requires immediate needle decompression and chest tube placement. Simple pneumothorax can often be managed with observation or tube thoracostomy.

Pericardial Tamponade: Unstable patients should undergo pericardiocentesis. Surgery may be necessary for a pericardial window.

Disposition

Admission: All patients with concerning presentations should be admitted to a monitored bed.

Discharge: Patients with a non-urgent diagnosis (e.g., chest wall pain, herpes zoster, dyspepsia) can be discharged with appropriate follow-up instructions. Any doubt about the diagnosis should warrant admission for observation.

Suggested Reading

1. Anderson JL, Adams CD, Antman EM, et al. ACC/AHA 2007 Guidelines for the management of unstable angina/non-ST elevation MI.

2. Anderson, J. L., Adams, C. D., Antman, E. M., et al. (2007). ACC/AHA 2007 Guidelines for the Management of Patients with Unstable Angina/Non-ST-Elevation Myocardial Infarction: A Report of the ACC/AHA Task Force on Practice Guidelines. Circulation, 116, e148.

3. Fesmire, F. M., Brown, M. D., Espinosa, J. A., et al. (2011). Critical Issues in the Evaluation and Management of Adult Patients Presenting to the Emergency Department with Suspected Pulmonary Embolism. Annals of Emergency Medicine, 57, 628-652.

4. Green, G. B., & Hill, P. M. (2011). Chest Pain: Cardiac or Not. In J. E. Tintinalli, J. S. Stapczynski, O. J. Ma, D. M. Cline, R. K. Cydulka, & G. D. Meckler (Eds.), Tintinalli's Emergency Medicine: A

Comprehensive Study Guide (7th ed., pp. 361-367). New York, NY: McGraw-Hill.

5. Swap, C. J., & Nagurney, J. T. (2005). Value and Limitations of Chest Pain History in the Evaluation of Patients with Acute Coronary Syndromes. JAMA, 294, 2623-2639.

## Chapter 14
## Acute Coronary Syndromes (ACS)

Key Points:

Acute coronary syndrome (ACS) should be considered in all patients presenting with chest pain or difficulty breathing.

Atypical presentations are common, particularly in women, elderly patients, and individuals with diabetes.

An urgent electrocardiogram (ECG) is essential for any patient suspected of ACS to quickly identify underlying cardiac issues.

Introduction

Acute Coronary Syndrome (ACS) includes a range of conditions such as unstable angina

(UA), non-ST-segment elevation myocardial infarction (NSTEMI), and ST-segment elevation myocardial infarction (STEMI). The differentiation between these conditions is based on clinical history, ECG findings, and cardiac biomarker levels. ACS is a leading cause of death globally, accounting for over 25% of all fatalities in the United States. Over five million patients each year present to U.S. emergency departments (EDs) with symptoms suggestive of ACS, though less than 10% are diagnosed with acute myocardial infarction (AMI). Unfortunately, between 2% and 4% of ACS patients are initially misdiagnosed and discharged from the ED, leading to significant morbidity and contributing to the leading cause of malpractice claims in the U.S.

The pathophysiology of ACS is rooted in an imbalance between coronary blood supply and myocardial demand. Atherosclerosis is the primary cause, beginning with the deposition of fatty streaks in the coronary arteries during adolescence, which progresses over time to form plaques. As these plaques enlarge, they progressively limit coronary blood flow and may cause angina. Eventually, plaque rupture and thrombus formation can lead to a sudden, complete occlusion of a coronary artery, resulting in an AMI.

Unstable Angina (UA): This is diagnosed clinically, and it does not exhibit pathognomonic ECG findings or elevated cardiac biomarkers. Symptoms typically include new or worsening angina, which may occur at rest or with minimal exertion.

NSTEMI and STEMI: Both are caused by a significant reduction or complete cessation of coronary blood flow. NSTEMI differs from STEMI in that cardiac biomarkers are elevated but no ST-segment elevation is seen. STEMI is characterized by ST-segment elevation on the ECG and a complete occlusion of a coronary artery, often resulting in transmural myocardial infarction.

Coronary Artery Anatomy

Understanding coronary artery anatomy is crucial for interpreting ECG findings and predicting clinical complications. The left coronary artery (LCA) branches into the left anterior descending artery (LAD) and left circumflex artery (LCX). The LAD supplies the anterior left ventricle and ventricular septum, while the LCX feeds the lateral and posterior parts of the heart. The right coronary artery (RCA) supplies the right side of the heart and the inferior left ventricle. It also perfuses the sinoatrial (SA) node in most individuals. The atrioventricular (AV) node receives blood from both the RCA and the LAD in most patients.

Risk Factors

Key risk factors for coronary artery disease (CAD) include age (especially over 40 years), male gender, postmenopausal women, hypertension, dyslipidemia, diabetes mellitus, smoking, family history of CAD, obesity, and a sedentary lifestyle. However, these risk factors are general trends and cannot definitively predict CAD in an individual patient. Around half of ACS patients lack identifiable risk factors other than age and gender.

Clinical Presentation

History: A detailed history is crucial for diagnosing ACS. Chest pain is the most common presenting symptom, often described as pressure or squeezing in the retrosternal or left chest region. Pain may radiate to the shoulder, arm, neck, or jaw. Patients may also experience associated symptoms such as nausea, sweating, shortness of breath, and palpitations. It is important to note that the intensity of pain does not necessarily correlate with the severity of the myocardial injury.

Non-chest pain symptoms, or "anginal equivalents," can present in up to a third of ACS patients. These may include shortness of breath, altered mental status, abdominal pain, or syncope, particularly in higher-risk groups such as the elderly, women, diabetics, and those with a history of substance abuse. Early detection in these groups is critical to improving outcomes.

Physical Examination: While there are no specific physical signs of ACS, monitoring vital signs is essential. Bradycardia may occur in cases of inferior wall ischemia due to vagal tone, while tachycardia can result from reduced stroke volume. Hypotension, especially in cases of cardiogenic shock, signifies a poor prognosis. Auscultation may reveal abnormal heart sounds, such as S3 or S4, or murmurs that may indicate complications such as papillary muscle infarction or ventricular septal perforation.

Diagnostic Studies

Electrocardiogram (ECG): A 12-lead ECG should be obtained immediately for any patient suspected of ACS. It helps to confirm the diagnosis and guide management, particularly for identifying STEMI. Prehospital ECGs are valuable for reducing treatment delays. It's important to understand that an ECG snapshot only provides a momentary view of myocardial electrical activity. Thus, repeat ECGs should be performed if the patient's clinical status changes.

ST-segment Elevation: Indicative of transmural infarction, particularly in leads corresponding to the affected area of the heart.

ST-segment Depression: Suggests active myocardial ischemia.

T-wave Abnormalities: Inverted or hyperacute T-waves may indicate ischemia.

Q-waves: Typically appear late in the course of an AMI and are not useful for acute decision-making.

Anatomical Considerations:

Anterior Wall Myocardial Infarction: Typically caused by occlusion of the LAD, affecting leads V2, V3, and V4.

Lateral Wall Myocardial Infarction: Often linked to the LCX, seen in leads I, aVL, V5, and V6.

Inferior Wall Myocardial Infarction: Commonly due to RCA occlusion, detected in leads II, III, and aVF.

Right Ventricular Infarction: Typically accompanies inferior wall infarctions, detected in leads V1 and V4R.

If a posterior wall infarction is suspected, consider obtaining a posterior ECG (leads V8 and V9). The presence of abnormal conduction patterns, including high-degree AV block or bundle branch blocks, warrants close monitoring and may indicate more severe infarction.

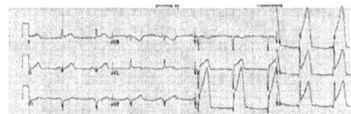

Figure 14-1. Anterior Wall Myocardial Infarction

This patient experienced a complete (100%) blockage of the left anterior descending artery.

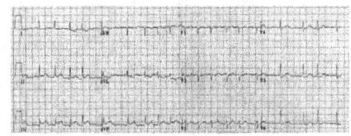

Figure 14-2. Inferior Wall Myocardial Infarction
ST segment elevations are observed in leads II, III, and aVF, with a more pronounced elevation in lead III, indicating potential right ventricular wall involvement.

Laboratory Analysis

Myocardial injury triggers the release of cardiac-specific enzymes into the bloodstream, which can be detected through serum analysis. Although patients exhibiting ECG signs of

STEMI do not need confirmatory testing with serum biomarkers and should receive immediate reperfusion therapy, serum markers are invaluable for diagnosing NSTEMI, particularly in cases with non-diagnostic ECGs. However, no single cardiac biomarker reliably excludes or confirms acute myocardial infarction (AMI) within the first 6 hours after symptom onset. Additionally, enzyme elevations may occur in non-ACS conditions such as myocarditis, decompensated heart failure, and acute pulmonary embolism.

Troponins (Tn), specifically the T and I subtypes, are the most specific biomarkers for myocardial damage and are considered the gold standard in diagnosing AMI. Elevated troponin levels typically become detectable within 3 hours of myocardial injury, peak at 12 hours, and remain elevated for 3 to 10 days. The severity of myocardial damage and associated mortality correlates with the magnitude of troponin elevation.

Creatine kinase (CK) is found in various muscle tissues, but the CK-MB subunit is more specific to myocardial injury. CK-MB levels rise within 4 to 6 hours of symptom onset, peak at 24 hours, and typically return to baseline within 2 to 3 days. Myoglobin is another biomarker used in the evaluation of AMI, though it has poor specificity despite being detectable within 1 to 2 hours of symptom onset, limiting its clinical utility.

Imaging

Chest X-rays should be obtained for all patients presenting with chest pain or shortness of breath. While radiographs cannot specifically diagnose acute coronary syndrome (ACS), they are essential for excluding other conditions. Classic findings of acute congestive heart failure (CHF) may be present in cases of ACS.

Medical Decision Making

An ECG should be performed immediately on presentation to identify patients with STEMI who require urgent reperfusion. Additionally, patients with cardiogenic shock, acutely decompensated CHF, ventricular arrhythmias, or severe symptoms unresponsive to medical therapy may also benefit from emergent percutaneous coronary intervention (PCI). In cases with non-diagnostic ECGs, cardiac marker testing should be conducted. Patients with elevated cardiac markers are likely experiencing NSTEMI and should be treated accordingly. Patients with negative biomarkers should be monitored with serial ECGs and biomarker tests. Risk stratification is essential, especially in patients over 65, those with multiple cardiovascular risk factors, significant coronary stenosis, ST-segment deviations on ECG, elevated cardiac markers, or a history of angina within the last 24 hours. Treatment should align with the patient's risk profile.

Treatment

Managing ACS requires swift, aggressive intervention, ideally in a facility equipped for resuscitation. Stabilize the patient's airway and circulatory status, and ensure continuous cardiac monitoring. Intravenous access should be established, and oxygen should be administered to maintain SpO2 ≥94%. Immediate treatment goals are to restore coronary blood flow and reduce myocardial oxygen demand, with further management tailored to STEMI or NSTEMI pathways.

Nitroglycerin is commonly used in ACS management for its ability to decrease myocardial oxygen demand, improve coronary perfusion, and exert mild antiplatelet effects. Administer sublingual nitroglycerin at a dose of 0.4 mg, repeating every 3 to 5 minutes as needed, provided the systolic blood pressure remains >100 mmHg. If pain persists after 3 to 5 doses, IV therapy should be initiated at 10–20 μg/min and titrated as necessary for pain relief. Careful monitoring is essential, especially in patients with right ventricular infarctions who may be prone to hypotension.

Morphine should be administered to patients with persistent pain despite nitroglycerin use. It reduces myocardial oxygen demand by decreasing vascular tone and limiting the catecholamine response. However, morphine should be avoided in hypotensive patients.

Antiplatelet Therapy is critical in ACS management. Aspirin (ASA) should be administered immediately at a dose of 160-325 mg of a non-enteric-coated version, with the first dose chewed for rapid absorption. Aspirin reduces mortality in STEMI patients by approximately 23%. Additional platelet inhibitors such as clopidogrel, prasugrel, and ticagrelor, which block the adenosine diphosphate (ADP) receptors, should be used in combination with aspirin. Clopidogrel is commonly employed, with a 600 mg loading dose recommended for STEMI patients undergoing PCI and a 300 mg dose for those undergoing thrombolysis or with NSTEMI. For patients over 75, a lower dose is recommended due to increased bleeding risks.

Glycoprotein IIb/IIIa inhibitors (abciximab, eptifibatide, tirofiban) block platelet aggregation and are used in patients undergoing PCI for ACS, although their use is associated with an increased risk of major bleeding.

Anticoagulation with unfractionated heparin (UFH) or low-molecular-weight heparin (LMWH) is indicated in all ACS patients without contraindications. LMWH (enoxaparin) is preferred for its predictable effect and lower bleeding risk, though UFH is recommended for patients undergoing PCI. Newer anticoagulants like fondaparinux and bivalirudin may have a role in select patient populations due to their similar efficacy and fewer bleeding complications.

Beta-Blockers should be administered to all ACS patients without contraindications.

Beta-blockers reduce myocardial oxygen demand by lowering heart rate, cardiac afterload, and contractility. Metoprolol is commonly used in a dose of 5 mg IV every 5 minutes for up to 3 doses, or as a 50 mg oral dose.

Reperfusion Therapy is essential for STEMI patients, with PCI preferred over thrombolysis due to reduced bleeding risks and better outcomes. PCI should be performed within 90 minutes of presentation, and thrombolysis should be initiated within 30 minutes. For patients with NSTEMI or unstable angina, early invasive PCI (within 24-48 hours) can reduce the risk of adverse outcomes.

Disposition

Admission: All patients with suspected ACS should be admitted for continuous monitoring and serial ECG and cardiac marker analysis. High-risk patients should be transferred to a critical care setting for early PCI.

Discharge: Patients at very low risk for ACS, such as young, healthy individuals with atypical symptoms, normal ECG, and negative biomarkers, can be safely discharged after a few hours of observation, with follow-up stress testing arranged.

Suggested Reading

1. Green, G., & Hill, P. (2011). Chest pain: Cardiac or not. In J. E. Tintinalli, J. S. Stapczynski, O. J. Ma, D. M. Cline, R. K. Cydulka, & G. D. Meckler (Eds.), Tintinalli's Emergency Medicine: A Comprehensive Study Guide (7th ed., pp. 361-367). New York, NY: McGraw-Hill.

2. Hollander, J., & Dierks, D. (2011). Acute coronary syndromes: Acute myocardial infarction. In J. E. Tintinalli, J. S. Stapczynski, O. J. Ma, D. M. Cline, R. K. Cydulka, & G. D. Meckler (Eds.), Tintinalli's Emergency Medicine: A

Comprehensive Study Guide (7th ed., pp. 367-383). New York, NY: McGraw-Hill.

## Chapter 15
## Congestive Heart Failure (CHF)

Key Points:

A normal ejection fraction (EF) does not rule out congestive heart failure (CHF), as CHF can result from both systolic and diastolic dysfunction.

Nitroglycerin is the preferred initial treatment because it decreases both preload and afterload, quickly alleviating symptoms.

Introduction

Congestive heart failure (CHF) is a leading cause of hospital admissions in patients over the age of 65 in the United States. Once symptomatic, about 35% of patients with CHF will die within 2 years, and over 60% will succumb within 6 years. Treatment costs annually exceed $27 billion, a figure that is expected to rise due to the aging population. CHF occurs when the heart cannot pump enough blood to meet the body's metabolic demands. As a result, pulmonary and systemic congestion develop due to the inability of the myocardium to manage venous return.

Common causes of CHF include myocardial infarction (MI), valvular diseases, cardiomyopathies, and long-standing uncontrolled hypertension. CHF can be classified into two subtypes based on pathophysiology:

1. Systolic heart failure occurs when myocardial injury impairs cardiac contractility, leading to a decrease in ejection fraction, often due to myocardial infarction.

2. Diastolic heart failure results from decreased ventricular compliance, limiting filling and

lowering cardiac output, commonly seen in conditions like left ventricular hypertrophy.

Pathophysiology of Acute Decompensated CHF

In acute decompensated CHF, reduced cardiac output triggers a compensatory increase in systemic vascular resistance (SVR) to maintain vital organ perfusion. However, this increase in SVR worsens cardiac output by elevating afterload, which further strains the myocardium. This leads to higher myocardial oxygen demand and increased left atrial and ventricular pressures, culminating in pulmonary edema and respiratory distress.

Precipitants of Decompensated CHF

Acute coronary syndrome (ACS), rapid atrial fibrillation, acute renal failure, and noncompliance with medications or diet are common precipitating factors. Additional causes to consider include pulmonary embolism, uncontrolled hypertension, anemia, thyroid dysfunction, and infections. Cardiotoxic drugs, such as alcohol, cocaine, and certain chemotherapeutic agents, should also be evaluated.

Clinical Presentation

History

Patients typically present with shortness of breath, which may occur during exertion or at rest. Orthopnea (dyspnea while lying flat) is common due to fluid redistribution from the lower extremities to the central circulation, increasing pulmonary capillary pressure and leading to pulmonary edema. Paroxysmal nocturnal dyspnea (PND) may also occur, where patients awaken with severe shortness of breath and feel the need to sit up or hang their legs over the side of the bed. Some patients may only report mild nocturnal cough as a sign of pulmonary congestion.

Peripheral edema, though common, is neither sensitive nor specific for CHF. Hepatic congestion can lead to right upper quadrant pain, which may be mistaken for biliary colic. A thorough review of systems should be performed, including questioning the patient about chest pain, palpitations, recent infections, and any changes or noncompliance with medications or diet.

Physical Examination

A rapid assessment of the patient's stability is essential. Vital signs should be monitored, and a focused physical exam should be performed. Observing the respiratory rate, checking pulse oximetry, looking for accessory muscle use, and determining if the patient can speak in full sentences can help assess the severity of respiratory distress. Tachycardia, narrow pulse pressure, and peripheral vasoconstriction are signs of decreased stroke volume and impaired cardiac output. Recognizing hypotension or signs of hypoperfusion is crucial, as these indicate cardiogenic shock.

A thorough examination for volume overload should be performed. Left ventricular failure often presents with pulmonary signs, such as inspiratory crackles, persistent cough, or a "cardiac wheeze." Right ventricular failure is associated with systemic congestion, including peripheral edema, jugular venous distention (JVD), and hepatojugular reflux (JVR). An S3 gallop is highly suggestive of decompensated heart failure, though it may be difficult to detect in an emergency setting.

Diagnostic Studies

Laboratory Studies

A complete blood count (CBC) should be obtained to check for anemia, and serum electrolytes and renal function should be assessed to rule out electrolyte imbalances like hyperkalemia, which can contribute to cardiac arrhythmias. Cardiac enzymes should be checked to rule out ACS as a precipitating factor. Elevated cardiac enzymes in CHF patients are associated with worse outcomes. Thyroid function tests are also important if thyroid dysfunction is suspected.

Brain natriuretic peptide (BNP) is a useful marker released during ventricular wall distension. Serum BNP levels can help differentiate CHF from pulmonary conditions like chronic obstructive pulmonary disease (COPD) or pneumonia. Levels below 100 ng/dL are highly predictive of the absence of CHF, while levels above 400 ng/dL are strongly indicative of decompensated CHF. Values between 100 and 400 ng/dL are inconclusive and may indicate other conditions like pulmonary embolism, cirrhosis, or renal failure.

Electrocardiogram (ECG)

An ECG should be obtained in all patients with suspected CHF to identify any new or old myocardial injury and arrhythmias. Signs of atrial or ventricular hypertrophy may also be observed.

Imaging

A chest X-ray (CXR) is essential for all CHF patients. Typical findings include cardiomegaly, bilateral pleural effusions, perihilar congestion, Kerley B lines, and vascular cephalization. However, a normal CXR does not exclude CHF, as radiographic changes can lag behind clinical symptoms. Echocardiography is often performed to assess ventricular function and rule out valvular disease. Point-of-care echocardiography may be used by skilled emergency providers to assess cardiac function in critically ill patients.

Medical Decision-Making

Immediate attention to respiratory distress is necessary. Patients with mild symptoms may only require supplemental oxygen, whereas those with moderate to severe distress may need ventilatory support, such as noninvasive positive pressure ventilation (NIPPV). NIPPV is beneficial in reducing the need for intubation in patients with acute CHF.

For patients who are hypotensive and showing signs of shock, inotropic and vasopressor support is essential. Dobutamine can provide inotropic support but may cause hypotension due to its vasodilatory effects. Dopamine or norepinephrine may be required to maintain blood pressure. Early cardiology consultation and emergent echocardiography are recommended for suspected ACS.

In patients with significant hypertension, vasodilators like nitroglycerin are the first-line treatment. Nitroglycerin reduces preload and afterload, improving cardiac output. It can be started with sublingual doses and increased as necessary for severe exacerbations. In cases where nitroglycerin is insufficient, nitroprusside may be used as a more potent vasodilator.

Treatment

The primary goals of treatment are symptom management, hemodynamic stabilization, and the reversal of precipitating factors. All patients with dyspnea and hypoxia should receive supplemental oxygen. NIPPV should be considered for patients who do not respond to oxygen therapy. It is contraindicated in those at risk for aspiration, with significant facial trauma, or who are unable to cooperate.

For patients with signs of cardiogenic shock, immediate hemodynamic support is required. Inotropic agents like dobutamine and vasopressors like dopamine or norepinephrine are often necessary to stabilize blood pressure. An aggressive search for the underlying precipitant, most commonly acute myocardial infarction, should be conducted. Early cardiology consultation is critical for further management.

For patients with marked hypertension, nitroglycerin is the initial treatment of choice. IV loop diuretics, such as furosemide, should be administered to reduce fluid overload and improve symptoms.

The medications used in the management of congestive heart failure (CHF) are varied, and their appropriate use is crucial for both symptom management and improving long-term outcomes. Below is a simplified analysis of these medications, detailing their mechanisms of action, dosing, adverse effects, and special considerations.

Vasodilators

Nitroglycerin is used to reduce preload (the volume of blood returning to the heart), making it easier for the heart to pump blood. It can be administered sublingually or intravenously. Sublingual nitroglycerin (0.4 mg) is given every 3-5 minutes as needed for symptoms, while the intravenous form is started at 25-50 mcg/min, with titration every 3-5 minutes based on patient response. The maximum dose is 400 mcg/min. Adverse effects include hypotension, tachycardia, and headaches, and its use should be limited to 24 hours due to the risk of tachyphylaxis (a reduction in effectiveness with prolonged use). Careful monitoring of blood pressure is required during administration.

Nitroprusside, which is administered intravenously, works by significantly reducing afterload (resistance against the heart's pumping action). The initial dose is 10-20 mcg/min, with titration every 5 minutes. Like nitroglycerin, the maximum dose is 400 mcg/min. This medication can also cause hypotension and, with prolonged use, cyanide toxicity, making it less ideal for long-term treatment. It's used mainly in critical care settings, requiring close monitoring of blood pressure.

Loop Diuretics

Furosemide is the most commonly used loop diuretic for CHF, administered intravenously at doses of 40-80 mg. If no diuresis (urine production) occurs, a re-dose may be given after 30 minutes, followed by every 12-hour dosing. The maximum recommended dose is 200 mg per dose. Its primary role is to promote sodium and water excretion, helping to relieve the symptoms of fluid overload. Electrolyte imbalances are a potential adverse effect, along with a risk of sulfa allergies and ototoxicity (hearing damage).

Bumetanide and Torsemide are alternative loop diuretics that are similar to furosemide but more potent. Bumetanide is administered at a dose of 1 mg IV, with the possibility of re-dosing every 2 hours. Torsemide, typically given at 10 mg IV, can also be re-dosed every 2 hours if needed. Both have the same adverse effects as furosemide, including electrolyte imbalances and ototoxicity, but are sometimes preferred for their more predictable and prolonged effects.

Ethacrynic Acid is another loop diuretic used primarily when a patient has a sulfa allergy, as it does not contain a sulfonamide group. It is typically given at 50 mg IV, with re-dosing possible after 8 hours. The main concern with this drug is the risk of ototoxicity and electrolyte disturbances, but it provides a suitable alternative for patients who cannot tolerate other diuretics.

Inotropes and Pressors

Dobutamine is an inotropic medication that primarily stimulates beta-1 receptors to improve heart contractility, though it also has some beta-2 and alpha effects. It is typically started at 2-5 mcg/kg/min, with titration to effect. Its maximum dose is 20 mcg/kg/min. It is often used in patients with cardiogenic shock (where the heart fails to pump blood effectively) to improve cardiac output. While it can be effective, it is limited by its vasodilatory effects, which can lower blood pressure, and it can cause tachycardia or arrhythmias.

Dopamine has dose-dependent effects: at low doses (3-5 mcg/kg/min), it primarily acts on dopaminergic receptors to increase renal blood flow. At higher doses, it stimulates beta-1 and beta-2 receptors to increase heart rate and contractility, and at very high doses, it can activate alpha-1 receptors to cause vasoconstriction. Like dobutamine, it is used in shock states and needs careful titration to avoid tachycardia or arrhythmias.

Norepinephrine acts mainly on alpha-1 receptors to cause vasoconstriction, raising blood pressure. It also has some beta-1 effects to improve heart contractility. It is administered at a starting dose of 2-5 mcg/min, titrated based on response, with a maximum dose of 30 mcg/min. Norepinephrine is crucial for managing shock and hypotension, though it can increase the risk of arrhythmias and cause tachycardia.

General Considerations and Notes

Blood Pressure Monitoring: For all vasodilators and inotropes/pressors, continuous monitoring of blood pressure is essential to avoid complications like hypotension.

Duration of Use: Many vasodilators and diuretics, particularly nitroglycerin and nitroprusside, are not suitable for long-term use due to risks like tachyphylaxis or toxicity. Inotropes, like dobutamine and dopamine, are typically used in acute settings or in combination with other agents to manage severe decompensation.

Electrolyte Imbalances: Loop diuretics, in particular, can cause electrolyte disturbances, so regular monitoring of sodium, potassium, and other electrolytes is necessary.

Sulfa Allergies: Furosemide, bumetanide, and torsemide are contraindicated in patients with sulfa allergies, while ethacrynic acid can be used as an alternative.

## Clinical Application and Management Strategy

In outpatient settings, CHF is primarily managed with ACE inhibitors and beta-blockers, both proven to reduce mortality in the long term. However, in acute exacerbations, these medications are usually avoided due to their effects on blood pressure. Oral furosemide is often used for symptomatic relief of fluid retention, although it doesn't offer survival benefits. For severe cases, medications are typically adjusted in a hospital setting, where echocardiography and careful medication titration can be done.

Patient Discharge: Asymptomatic patients with stable vital signs and no acute underlying issues may be safely discharged. Education on medication compliance, diet, and the importance of follow-up care is crucial to prevent readmission, as many patients are readmitted within six months.

Hospital Admission: Most patients experiencing acute CHF exacerbations require hospitalization for monitoring, especially in the presence of underlying causes such as infection or ischemia. Proper titration of medications like diuretics, vasodilators, and inotropes ensures optimal outcomes.

Key Takeaways:

Effective management of CHF involves a combination of vasodilators, diuretics, and inotropes/pressors, tailored to the severity of the patient's condition. Close monitoring of blood pressure, electrolytes, and renal function is essential, particularly when using agents like diuretics and inotropes. These medications are mainly used in the acute setting, and long-term CHF management includes ACE inhibitors, beta-blockers, and proper lifestyle modifications.

Suggested Reading

1. Collins S, Storrow AB, Kirk JD, et al. "Beyond Pulmonary Edema: Challenges in Diagnosing, Risk Stratifying, and Treating Acute Heart Failure in the Emergency Department." Annals of Emergency Medicine. 2008;51:45.

2. Heart Failure Society of America, Lindenfeld J, Albert NM, et al. "HFSA 2010 Comprehensive Heart Failure Practice Guidelines." Journal of Cardiac Failure. 2010;16:e1.

3. Peacock WF. "Congestive Heart Failure and Acute Pulmonary Edema." In: Tintinalli JE, Stapczynski JS, Ma OJ, Cline DM, Cydulka RK, Meckler GD, eds. Tintinalli's Emergency Medicine: A Comprehensive Study Guide, 7th ed. New York, NY: McGraw-Hill, 2011:405-414.

4. Silvers SM, Howell JM, Kosowsky JM, et al. "Clinical Policy: Key Issues in Evaluating and Managing Adult Patients

with Acute Heart Failure Syndromes Presenting to the Emergency Department." Annals of Emergency Medicine. 2007;49.

# Chapter 16
# Dysrhythmias

Key Points

Initial Management

Immediately assess and address airway, breathing, and circulation (ABCs), provide oxygen as needed, secure intravenous (IV) access, and initiate continuous cardiac monitoring.

Stability Assessment

Quickly differentiate between stable and unstable patients. Unstable presentations require urgent intervention.

Introduction

Recognizing dysrhythmias is critical for emergency physicians, as these cases are common and may lead to rapid hemodynamic compromise. Dysrhythmias are clinically categorized as stable or unstable, depending on the adequacy of end-organ perfusion (e.g., systemic hypotension, cardiac ischemia, pulmonary edema, altered mental status). They are further classified by heart rate into bradydysrhythmias (HR <60 bpm) and tachydysrhythmias (HR >100 bpm). Additionally, atrioventricular (AV) blocks can present at any heart rate, resulting from disrupted electrical conduction between the sinoatrial (SA) node, AV node, and ventricles.

Understanding the normal cardiac rhythm and conduction pathway is essential. Normal rhythm begins at the SA node, then moves through the atria to the AV node, which serves as the "gatekeeper" for ventricular conduction. From the AV node, impulses travel through the bundle of His, branch bundles, and Purkinje fibers, finally reaching the ventricular myocardium.

ECG Considerations: Perform a 12-lead ECG on stable patients and investigate possible causes, such as acute coronary syndrome (ACS), electrolyte imbalances, toxicity, or medication effects.

ECG Components

A standard ECG consists of a P wave, QRS complex, and T wave. The P wave indicates atrial depolarization, followed by the PR interval (120-200 ms). The QRS complex, which represents ventricular depolarization, is normally under 100 ms. Abnormal intraventricular conduction appears as a widened QRS (>100 ms). The ST segment reflects the plateau phase of ventricular depolarization and is typically isoelectric, while the T wave represents ventricular repolarization.

Bradydysrhythmias: Result from suppressed sinus node activity or blocked electrical conduction, often due to structural heart damage, elevated vagal tone, medications, or electrolyte disturbances (e.g., hyperkalemia).

Tachydysrhythmias: Caused by increased automaticity from the SA node or an ectopic source, originating from either atrial or ventricular areas. Supraventricular tachycardia (SVT) often involves re-entry loops in the AV node or accessory pathways.

Classifying Dysrhythmias

Wide QRS complexes indicate ventricular depolarization outside the normal conduction system, while narrow complexes originate from or above the AV node and utilize normal pathways. Dysrhythmia severity and management vary widely. For example, atrial fibrillation (AF) is common and can range from asymptomatic to requiring immediate intervention, while ventricular fibrillation is often fatal without prompt action.

Assessment Steps: Determine hemodynamic stability, assess hypoperfusion signs (e.g., hypotension, chest pain, altered mental status, or heart failure), classify rhythm rate as slow or fast, examine QRS morphology (narrow vs. wide), check rhythm regularity, and evaluate for AV conduction block.

Dysrhythmia Types by Rhythm Characteristics

Narrow Complex:

Fast: Atrial fibrillation, atrial flutter, SVT

Slow: Sinus bradycardia, junctional escape rhythm

Wide Complex:

Fast: Ventricular tachycardia (VT), AF, or flutter with aberrant conduction

Slow: Hyperkalemia, third-degree heart block

Clinical Presentation

History

Unstable patients may not provide a detailed history. Obtain critical information from family, friends, or emergency medical services (EMS). For stable patients, ask about prior dysrhythmic episodes, current medications, illicit drug use, symptom onset, and relevant medical history (e.g., Wolff-Parkinson-White syndrome). Older patients with coronary artery disease (CAD) are at risk for pathological bradydysrhythmias, while sinus tachycardia in CAD or valvular disease often has a pathological cause.

Physical Examination

Assess hemodynamic stability, repeatedly monitor vital signs, and palpate pulses to match with cardiac monitor rhythm. Look for end-organ hypoperfusion (e.g., weak peripheral pulses, rales, altered mental state). Certain findings, like a goiter in thyrotoxicosis or an AV fistula in dialysis patients, may indicate specific underlying causes.

Diagnostic Studies

Electrocardiogram (ECG): For suspected dysrhythmias, initiate continuous cardiac monitoring and obtain a 12-lead ECG unless immediate interventions, like cardioversion or pacing, are needed. Assess heart rate, rhythm regularity, and classify the QRS complex as narrow (<100 ms) or wide.

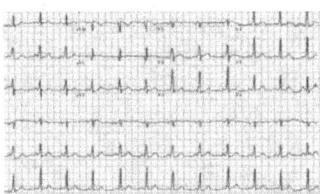

Figure 16-1. Wolf-Parkinson-White Syndrome

Laboratory Testing

To identify potential causes of dysrhythmia, conduct a complete blood count to check for anemia and a metabolic panel to detect electrolyte imbalances. If there's suspicion of cardiac ischemia, assess cardiac enzyme levels. For patients on digoxin, measure serum digoxin levels. In cases of tachycardia with potential risk factors, consider D-dimer testing to evaluate for pulmonary embolism and thyroid function tests to rule out thyroid disease.

Imaging

A chest X-ray should be performed to check for indications of congestive heart failure or structural heart disease, such as valvulopathy.

Clinical Decision-Making

Approaching dysrhythmia assessment systematically, begin with a quick evaluation of the patient's hemodynamic stability. For those who are unstable, provide immediate intervention. For stable cases, perform a 12-lead ECG, optionally with a rhythm strip, to identify the specific rhythm and guide treatment choices. Therapeutic strategies may include vagal maneuvers, antiarrhythmic medications, or electrical interventions like defibrillation, cardioversion, or pacing.

Bradydysrhythmias

In patients with bradydysrhythmias, first check if each QRS complex is preceded by a P wave and whether the PR interval remains constant. A regular, slow rhythm with a consistent PR interval typically suggests sinus bradycardia or sinus bradycardia with first-degree AV block (characterized by a PR interval over 200 milliseconds) and usually doesn't require urgent intervention. Investigate and address any underlying causes.

When there are more P waves than QRS complexes, suspect higher-degree AV blocks, like second- or third-degree AV blocks.

Second-degree AV blocks are categorized into Mobitz type I and type II:

Type I (Wenckebach): The PR interval progressively lengthens until an atrial impulse fails to conduct to the ventricles, leading to a dropped QRS complex. A shortening interval between R waves is typical.

Type II: The PR interval remains constant, but some P waves are not conducted to the ventricles, resulting in intermittent QRS drops. Type II is often more severe and requires close monitoring and, in many cases, intervention.

In a third-degree (complete) heart block, the atria and ventricles beat independently, and the QRS complexes (escape beats) can appear narrow (junctional) or wide (ventricular), depending on the origin (Figure 16-3).

Additional Bradycardias

Two other types of bradycardias are notable:

Junctional Bradycardia: A slow, regular rhythm with narrow QRS complexes and absent or abnormal P waves, usually caused by medications (e.g., beta-blockers).

Idioventricular Rhythm: Originating in the ventricles, this slow rhythm appears as wide QRS complexes (20-40 bpm) without discernible P waves.

Tachydysrhythmias

For stable tachycardia patients, assess rhythm regularity and distinguish between narrow (supraventricular) and wide (ventricular) QRS complexes. Fast, narrow, and regular rhythms commonly include sinus tachycardia, atrial flutter, and supraventricular tachycardia (SVT). Techniques such as vagal maneuvers or adenosine administration can slow the heart rate, aiding in rhythm identification and sometimes resolving SVT. Although adenosine is generally safe for narrow QRS complexes, it should be used cautiously in patients with pre-excitation syndromes (e.g., WPW). Assume any wide complex tachycardia is ventricular tachycardia (VT) unless otherwise proven, especially in elderly patients with cardiac disease.

Differentiation in Supraventricular Rhythms

Sinus Tachycardia: Displays a P wave before each QRS complex and regular R-R intervals, often secondary to conditions like fever, pain, or hypovolemia.

Atrial Flutter: Characterized by a "sawtooth" pattern of flutter waves with regular R-R intervals, usually at a rate of ~150 bpm due to 2:1 conduction through the AV node.

Atrial Fibrillation (AF): Irregular R-R intervals without discernible P waves. Distinguish AF from multifocal atrial tachycardia (MAT), where variable P wave morphologies and R-R intervals are present.

## Management of Wide-Complex Tachycardias

Wide-complex tachycardias, often requiring urgent intervention, may include VT and ventricular fibrillation (VF). VT is marked by rates above 120 bpm, wide QRS complexes, and absent P waves. A unique type, torsades de pointes, features a twisting QRS axis due to repolarization abnormalities. VF, a non-perfusing rhythm, demands immediate defibrillation.

### Treatment Approach

Start by ensuring patient airway, breathing, and circulation, provide supplemental oxygen, secure IV access, and monitor cardiac rhythm. Tailor treatment based on stability and rhythm type.

### Bradydysrhythmias

For unstable bradycardia, administer IV atropine (0.5–1.0 mg) and consider epinephrine (0.3–0.5 mg) if unresponsive. Transcutaneous pacing should be initiated, with transvenous pacing as a next step if needed. For Mobitz Type II and third-degree blocks, initiate transcutaneous pacing immediately if unstable, and consult cardiology for possible ICU admission and pacemaker placement.

Tachydysrhythmias

For unstable tachydysrhythmias, perform synchronized cardioversion or defibrillation as appropriate. In AF and atrial flutter, manage the ventricular rate using agents like beta-blockers or diltiazem, monitoring for hypotension. For SVT, attempt vagal maneuvers and escalate adenosine administration if needed.

For stable VT, consider antiarrhythmic agents such as amiodarone or procainamide. Torsades de pointes is treated with IV magnesium sulfate to shorten the QT interval.

Disposition

Admission: Patients with significant dysrhythmias showing signs of organ hypoperfusion or ischemia should be admitted to an intensive care setting. Those at high risk for recurrence or needing medication adjustments should be placed in a monitored setting.

Discharge: Patients who respond well to ED treatment, including those with AVNRT or well-controlled AF/flutter, may be discharged with appropriate follow-up if they remain asymptomatic.

Recommended Reading

1. Knight, J., & Sarko, J. "Ventricular Dysrhythmias." In Cardiac Emergencies, edited by W.F. Peacock and B.R. Tiffany, New York, NY: McGraw-Hill, 2006, pp. 219–236.

2. Moffa, D.A. "Cardiac Conduction Blocks." In Cardiac Emergencies, edited by W.F. Peacock and B.R. Tiffany, New York, NY: McGraw-Hill, 2006, pp. 250–268.

3. Piktel, J.S. "Cardiac Rhythm Disturbances." In Tintinalli's Emergency Medicine: A Comprehensive Study Guide, 7th ed., edited by J.E. Tintinalli, J.S. Stapczynski, O.J. Ma, D.M. Clince, R.K. Cydulka, and G.D. Meckler, New York, NY: McGraw-Hill, 2011, pp. 129–154.

4. Walters, D.J., & Dunbar, L.M. "Atrial Arrhythmias." In Cardiac Emergencies, edited by W.F. Peacock and B.R. Tiffany, New York, NY: McGraw-Hill, 2006, pp. 237–249.

## Chapter 17
## Aortic Dissection

Key Points

Always suspect aortic dissection in patients with sudden chest or thoracic back pain.

Immediate control of heart rate and blood pressure is essential in patients highly suspected of having aortic dissection, even before diagnostic imaging is confirmed.

Introduction

Aortic dissection, although rare, is a serious and often life-threatening condition. It affects approximately 6,000 to 10,000 individuals annually in the United States. Higher incidence is observed in men and older adults, with around 75% of cases occurring in patients aged 40 to 70.

Younger patients with this condition often have underlying connective tissue diseases. Notably, in women under 40, about 50% of aortic dissections develop in the third trimester or early postpartum period.

Risk factors for acute aortic dissection include chronic hypertension, bicuspid aortic valve, coarctation of the aorta, and inherited connective tissue disorders, such as Marfan and Ehlers-Danlos syndromes. Vascular inflammatory conditions like Takayasu arteritis and giant cell arteritis may also increase risk.

The pathology of aortic dissection involves an intimal tear in the aortic wall. High blood pressure propels blood through this tear into the media layer, causing the intima to separate from the adventitia and creating a false lumen. This false lumen can extend distally (antegrade), proximally (retrograde), or both. Occasionally, the false lumen ruptures, resulting in sudden hemodynamic collapse. Most dissections begin in the ascending aorta (65%), the aortic arch

(10%), or just distal to the ligamentum (20%). According to the Stanford classification system, Type A dissections involve the ascending aorta, while Type B dissections are restricted to the descending aorta, originating distal to the left subclavian artery.

Clinical Presentation

History

Typically, acute thoracic aortic dissection manifests in a middle-aged male (aged 55–65) with chronic hypertension. The patient often experiences an abrupt, severe chest pain described as "sharp" or "tearing," which may radiate to the interscapular region. Although less common, atypical presentations occur and may include intermittent symptoms or isolated syncope without chest pain. Patients often report visceral symptoms such as nausea, vomiting, diaphoresis, and pallor.

Physical Examination

Focus on the patient's general appearance and vital signs, as acute dissections frequently produce distress and a visibly uncomfortable appearance. Check for discrepancies in blood pressure across both arms; although a difference of over 20 mmHg raises suspicion for dissection, its absence does not rule out the condition. Cardiac examination should include auscultation for diastolic murmurs, which may suggest aortic regurgitation. Additional examinations should include checking for signs of pericardial tamponade and performing a neurologic exam to identify any signs of hemiplegia or paraplegia.

Diagnostic Studies

Laboratory Tests No specific lab tests can definitively diagnose aortic dissection. However, a d-dimer assay shows high sensitivity (94–99%) but should not be solely relied upon. Routine lab tests (CBC, metabolic panel, troponin I) are used mainly to rule out other conditions or identify complications associated with aortic dissection.

Imaging

A chest radiograph is often the first imaging test used, with 80–90% of cases showing abnormalities, such as an abnormal aortic contour or widened mediastinum. For a more definitive diagnosis, CT angiography is typically employed, offering high sensitivity (100%) and specificity (98%). This imaging can help distinguish between ascending and descending dissections and provide insights into alternative diagnoses. Transthoracic echocardiography (TTE) and transesophageal echocardiography (TEE) are useful, particularly when a patient is too unstable for CT. While TTE's sensitivity is only around 59.3%, TEE's sensitivity is 98%. MRI is highly sensitive but often impractical due to limited availability and time constraints in emergency settings.

Medical Decision Making

Obtaining a detailed patient history is crucial in suspected cases of aortic dissection. Consider differential diagnoses, including myocardial infarction, pulmonary embolism, abdominal aortic aneurysm, and tension pneumothorax. A patient's pain characteristics, risk factors, and rapid bedside imaging findings (portable chest X-ray, ultrasound) will help guide diagnosis and prioritize interventions based on patient stability.

Treatment

The initial management of acute aortic dissection involves promptly reducing heart rate and blood pressure to minimize shear forces on the aortic wall and prevent further propagation of the dissection. Target heart rate is below 60 bpm, and systolic blood pressure should be kept between 90 and 120 mmHg. Administer pain relief with opiates to reduce sympathetic stimulation.

Beta-blockers are the preferred initial treatment to reduce both heart rate and blood pressure.

Esmolol, due to its rapid onset and short duration, is frequently used. Start with a loading dose of 500 mcg/kg, followed by a continuous infusion at 50 mcg/kg/min. If adequate control is not achieved within 5 minutes, repeat the loading dose and increase the infusion rate. In cases of persistent hypertension, introduce an arterial vasodilator like nitroprusside as an adjunct therapy.

Suggested Reading

1. Klompas, M. "Does This Patient Have an Acute Thoracic Aortic Dissection?" Journal of the American Medical Association, vol. 287, 2002, pp. 2262–2272.

2. Upadhye, S., and K. Schiff. "Acute Aortic Dissection in the Emergency Department: Diagnostic Challenges and Evidence-Based Management."

Emergency Medicine Clinics of North America, vol. 30, 2012, pp. 307–327.

3. Wittels, K. "Aortic Emergencies." Emergency Medicine Clinics of North America, vol. 29, 2011, pp. 789–800.

## Chapter 18
## Hypertensive Emergencies: Summary and Analysis

Key Points

Hypertension is frequently encountered in emergency departments; however, the occurrence of hypertension leading to acute organ damage, necessitating immediate intervention, is rare.

A patient's history and physical examination are crucial in evaluating cases of severe hypertension.

Introduction

Hypertension impacts approximately 30% of adults in the U.S., making it one of the most prevalent medical conditions. Among those affected, nearly 75% have poorly controlled blood pressure (above 140/90 mmHg), and less than half adhere to their prescribed medication regimen. Despite these statistics, fewer than 1% of all hypertension cases progress to hypertensive emergencies.

Patients with a systolic BP of ≥180 mmHg or a diastolic BP of ≥110 mmHg are classified as experiencing severe hypertension. In these instances, it is critical to differentiate between a hypertensive emergency and a hypertensive urgency, as they require distinctly different approaches. Hypertensive emergencies are characterized by significant elevations in blood pressure, coupled with active end-organ damage, impacting organs such as the brain, heart, kidneys, and eyes. In contrast, hypertensive urgency is a severe increase in BP without acute end-organ dysfunction.

The underlying mechanism in hypertensive emergencies typically involves a rapid rise in systemic vascular resistance due to excessive vasoconstrictor release, which leads to endothelial injury and dysfunction, vascular permeability, and local blood clot formation. This cascade can ultimately result in tissue hypoperfusion and subsequent organ dysfunction.

Most individuals presenting with a hypertensive emergency have a prior history of hypertension. It is vital to consider chronic hypertension's impact on cerebral circulation when determining blood pressure management goals. Overly aggressive BP reduction can risk hypoperfusion and potential ischemia within the central nervous system (CNS).

Clinical Presentation

History A prompt evaluation of patients with severe hypertension should prioritize identifying any signs of end-organ damage. Key symptoms to assess include:

Chest or back pain, shortness of breath, and decreased urine output.

Neurological signs such as headache, weakness, confusion, or vision changes.

Specific Conditions and Presentations

Hypertensive Encephalopathy: Altered mental state, headache, seizures, vomiting, and vision changes, with mental states ranging from drowsiness to coma.

Intracranial Hemorrhage: Sudden headache, focal neurological deficits, and altered mental status.

Acute Pulmonary Edema: Shortness of breath, orthopnea, hemoptysis, and chest pain.

Acute Coronary Syndrome (ACS): Often presents with chest pain but may also include subtle signs of heart failure.

Aortic Dissection: Severe tearing chest or back pain with possible neurologic deficits and abdominal pain.

Acute Renal Failure: Symptoms may be subtle but often include hematuria, reduced urine output, and leg swelling from fluid retention.

Physical Examination

Ensure BP readings are accurate, considering cuff size and patient anatomy.

Conduct a thorough exam focused on neurological, cardiac, pulmonary, and abdominal assessments.

Notable findings may include signs of hypertensive encephalopathy, such as retinal hemorrhages and papilledema, or, in cases of intracranial hemorrhage, focal deficits and meningeal signs.

ACS signs may include diaphoresis and evidence of heart failure, while aortic dissection might show unequal pulses or a new aortic murmur.

Diagnostic Studies

Electrocardiogram (ECG): Useful for detecting cardiac ischemia in suspected ACS cases.

Laboratory Tests: Include urinalysis (for hematuria and proteinuria), renal function tests (BUN and creatinine), pregnancy testing in reproductive-aged women, and cardiac biomarkers (troponin) for chest pain or shortness of breath.

Imaging: A CT scan of the head can identify hypertensive encephalopathy or intracranial hemorrhage, while a chest X-ray and CT angiography may help diagnose flash pulmonary edema or aortic dissection.

Medical Decision Making

Promptly identify cases of hypertensive emergency, such as hypertensive encephalopathy, intracranial hemorrhage, pulmonary edema, ACS, aortic dissection, and renal injury. This involves using clinical history, physical examination, and diagnostic studies to confirm organ damage and guide treatment.

Treatment

Hypertensive emergencies require immediate BP control to prevent further organ damage, targeting a 20% reduction in mean arterial pressure (MAP) within the first 30 minutes. This is best achieved using intravenous medications tailored to the specific clinical scenario (Table 18-2). However, aortic dissection necessitates a faster reduction, aiming for a systolic BP below 100 mmHg and a heart rate under 60 bpm. Optimal BP targets for intracranial hemorrhage remain controversial, and cautious BP reduction is advised.

Recommended Reading

1. Cline, D. M., & Machado, A. J. "Systemic and Pulmonary Hypertension." In Tintinalli's Emergency Medicine: A Comprehensive Study Guide, edited by J. E. Tintinalli, J. S. Stapczynski, O. J. Ma, D. M. Cline, R. K. Cydulka, and G. D. Meckler, 7th edition, 441-448. New York, NY: McGraw-Hill, 2011.

2. Marik, P. E., & Rivera, R. "Hypertensive Emergencies: An Update." Current Opinion in Critical Care 17 (2011): 569.

3. Marik, P. E., & Varon, J. "Hypertensive Crisis: Challenges and Management." Chest 131 (2007): 1949.

225

# Chapter 19
# Syncope Management

Key Considerations

1. Immediate Monitoring and Assessment

For all patients presenting with syncope, ensure they are placed on a cardiac monitor, obtain a bedside glucose test urgently, and start continuous pulse oximetry.

2. Detailed History Collection

Gather a comprehensive history of the episode, including details from bystanders such as family members or emergency personnel, to capture critical context.

Introduction

Syncope refers to a temporary loss of consciousness paired with an inability to sustain posture, followed by a quick, spontaneous recovery. In the U.S., about 12-48% of people will experience syncope at some point, representing 1-3% of emergency department (ED) visits and 1-6% of hospital admissions. The causes range from benign to immediately life-threatening, and it is often challenging to determine the exact cause in the ED. However, a thorough patient history, physical examination, and selective testing can help identify high-risk cases needing hospitalization and further evaluation.

Syncope typically arises due to reduced blood flow to the brain, particularly the reticular activating system or both cerebral hemispheres, often due to low systemic blood pressure or direct reduction in central nervous system (CNS) blood flow (e.g., from subarachnoid hemorrhage). The resultant reduction in cerebral blood flow causes unconsciousness and loss of posture, followed by a reflexive sympathetic response that normalizes blood flow and restores consciousness. Near-syncope refers to feeling faint without actual unconsciousness and is evaluated similarly to full syncope.

Syncope is generally categorized by cause: neural-mediated (reflex), orthostatic, cerebrovascular, and cardiac.

1. Neurally Mediated (Reflex) Syncope: Also known as vasovagal syncope, this occurs from excessive parasympathetic activity, often in reaction to stress, leading to bradycardia and vasodilation that lower cardiac output and brain perfusion. Symptoms often include feelings of dizziness, warmth, and lightheadedness. Triggering situations include coughing, urination, or defecation, which raise vagal tone.

2. Orthostatic Syncope: Caused by a temporary blood pressure drop upon sitting or standing up, often due to volume depletion (e.g., from

dehydration or blood loss) or autonomic dysfunction, particularly in older adults prone to decreased sympathetic responses and medication side effects.

3. Cerebrovascular Syncope: Rarely, cerebrovascular issues like a sudden increase in intracranial pressure (e.g., from a subarachnoid hemorrhage) reduce cerebral perfusion, causing syncope. These cases may present with prolonged recovery periods, helping differentiate them from other causes.

4. Cardiac Syncope: Resulting from structural heart issues or arrhythmias that impair cardiac output, cardiac syncope can occur without warning, often during or right after exertion, as seen in hypertrophic cardiomyopathy or aortic stenosis. Cardiac-related syncope carries a higher risk, with a 1-year mortality rate of 18-33%.

## Clinical Presentation

### History

A thorough history is essential and may identify the cause in up to 40% of cases. Document all events preceding, during, and following the episode, gathering details from witnesses if possible. Look for warning symptoms like headache (suggestive of subarachnoid hemorrhage), chest pain (possibly myocardial infarction or aortic dissection), and abdominal or back pain (indicating potential ruptured aneurysm or ectopic pregnancy). Medical history, especially cardiovascular conditions, and medication review are critical, as certain drugs can predispose patients to orthostatic syncope or arrhythmias.

Signs of nausea, sweating, or dizziness, or the occurrence of syncope after moving to an upright position, may indicate benign vasovagal or orthostatic causes. Sudden syncope without warning or during exertion suggests cardiac causes. A prolonged recovery period may point to cerebrovascular issues.

Physical Examination

Always assess vital signs upon triage and repeat if abnormal. Measure blood pressure in both arms to check for aortic dissection, and consider orthostatic vital signs. Important findings include a drop of ≥20 mmHg in systolic BP or standing systolic BP ≤90 mmHg, which may indicate volume depletion or medication effects. Conduct a detailed cardiovascular and neurological examination, listening for arrhythmias or murmurs indicating structural heart issues. Perform a stool guaiac test to detect gastrointestinal bleeding if warranted.

Diagnostic Studies

Laboratory Tests

Routine lab work is based on specific findings from the history and physical examination. Perform a rapid glucose test for patients with altered consciousness. For women of childbearing age, conduct a urine pregnancy test. In patients with bleeding history or positive stool guaiac, check a complete blood count. Electrolyte imbalances should be ruled out in suspected cardiac dysrhythmias, and cardiac markers may be necessary for patients with chest pain or dyspnea.

Electrocardiogram (ECG)

An ECG should be obtained for all patients with syncope, although it rarely ($\leq 5\%$) identifies the cause directly. Look for abnormalities such as signs of ischemia, conduction delays, ectopy, arrhythmias, or evidence of cardiomyopathy.

Imaging

Routine CT of the head is generally unnecessary unless history and physical examination indicate a cerebrovascular cause. Indications include headache, focal neurological symptoms, or extended recovery post-syncope. Chest X-rays can help assess for cardiomegaly, aortic dissection, or heart failure, especially if syncope is sudden and lacks a prodrome or is accompanied by chest pain.

Medical Decision-Making

Follow a structured approach for managing syncope patients. Start with a broad differential diagnosis, prioritizing life-threatening causes. Evaluate initial vitals and perform bedside glucose testing. Use ECG and cardiac monitoring, followed by a comprehensive history (including witness accounts), medical review, and detailed cardiovascular and neurological exams. Tailor laboratory and imaging studies based on these findings. After ruling out immediate dangers, focus on benign causes, recognizing that the exact cause may remain unidentified in the ED.

Treatment

First, assess hemodynamic stability and provide supportive care. Ensure IV access, administer oxygen as needed, and conduct continuous cardiac monitoring. For low glucose levels, provide dextrose. Subsequent treatment focuses on the cause:

Cardiac Syncope: Address cardiac dysrhythmias per ACLS guidelines, avoid preload-reducing agents like nitroglycerin in cases of hypertrophic cardiomyopathy or aortic stenosis, and manage pulmonary embolism or aortic dissection if suspected.

Cerebrovascular Syncope: If subarachnoid hemorrhage is suspected, obtain an urgent CT scan and manage accordingly.

Orthostatic Syncope: Start isotonic saline for volume resuscitation, especially if internal bleeding is suspected, and avoid medications contributing to hypotension.

Reflex/Vasovagal Syncope: Usually no further treatment is needed beyond identifying and managing triggers.

## Disposition

Admission Criteria: Hospitalize patients with risk factors or clinical findings suggestive of cardiac syncope. Criteria include age over 45, abnormal vital signs (e.g., hypoxia, systolic BP <90 mmHg), ECG abnormalities, history of heart disease, low hematocrit (<30%), abnormal physical findings, positive stool guaiac, exertional or unprovoked syncope, or symptoms like shortness of breath.

Discharge: Patients at low cardiac risk (normal physical exam, no history of CAD/CHF, normal ECG, age <45) may be discharged if non-cardiac threats are excluded. Follow-up tests, such as Holter monitoring or tilt-table testing, may be arranged in an outpatient setting.

Suggested Reading

1. Chen L, Benditt D, et al. Management of syncope in adults: An update. Mayo Clinic Proceedings. 2008; 83:1280-1293.

2. Huff J, Decker W, et al. Clinical policy: Critical issues in the evaluation and management of patients presenting to the emergency department with syncope. Annals of Emergency Medicine. 2007; 49:431-444.

3. Quinn J. Syncope. In: Tintinalli JE, Stapczynski JS, Ma OJ, Cline DM, Cydulka RK, Meckler GD, editors. Tintinalli's Emergency Medicine: A Comprehensive Study Guide. 7th ed. New York, NY: McGraw-Hill, 2011. pp. 399-405.

4. Quinn J, McDermott M, et al. Prospective validation of the San Francisco rule to predict patients with serious outcomes. Annals of Emergency Medicine. 2006; 47:448-454.

## Chapter 20
## Dyspnea: An Overview of Assessment and Management

Key Points

Prioritize identifying any immediate life-threatening conditions.

Address three critical questions when dealing with patients in moderate to severe respiratory distress.

Use a systematic, anatomic approach for diagnosing the underlying causes of dyspnea.

Introduction

Dyspnea, commonly known as "shortness of breath," refers to the sensation of labored or difficult breathing, often caused by a physiological disturbance. It manifests as a feeling of breathlessness or "air hunger" and is usually associated with difficulty breathing. Tachypnea, which is rapid breathing, may or may not accompany dyspnea. Hyperventilation, characterized by excessive ventilation beyond metabolic needs, often results from psychological triggers such as anxiety.

From a clinical perspective, dyspnea typically arises from an issue in oxygen delivery to tissues. The problem may originate at various levels—starting from the airway, where obstruction can occur, to the cellular level, where the inability to offload oxygen occurs. A step-by-step diagnostic approach, beginning at the airway and extending to tissue-level issues, can help identify the specific cause. However, in severe cases of respiratory distress, treatment should be initiated immediately, even if full diagnostics are not complete.

Clinical Presentation

In the initial assessment of dyspnea severity, ask the following three questions:

1. Does the patient need immediate intubation?

Do not delay treatment in cases of severe respiratory distress. Indicators for immediate intubation include:

Inability to oxygenate (can result in anoxic injury, particularly to the brain).

Inability to ventilate (leading to carbon dioxide buildup and acidosis, which may compromise cardiac function).

Inability to protect the airway (due to factors like brain injury or mechanical obstruction).

2. Is respiratory distress rapidly reversible?

Identifying rapidly reversible causes can prevent further deterioration. Conditions such as:

Hypoxia: Managed with supplemental oxygen.

Bronchospasm: Treated with beta-agonists, steroids, or epinephrine.

Hypertensive pulmonary edema: Managed with nitrates or diuretics.

Pneumothorax: Treated by needle decompression or chest tube placement.

Allergic reactions: Treated with steroids, epinephrine, or antihistamines.

3. What is the patient's physiologic reserve?

Assess the patient's ability to maintain adequate breathing under stress. Consider the patient's age, overall health, exercise tolerance, and any pre-existing conditions that might impact respiratory function. If the patient is stable, allow time for therapy to take effect and reassess frequently. In patients with limited reserves or those showing signs of respiratory fatigue, intubation may be necessary sooner.


History Taking:

Exertional Dyspnea: Is the shortness of breath related to activity or physical exertion?

Positional Dyspnea: Does the patient experience difficulty breathing when lying down? This may suggest conditions like congestive heart failure (CHF) or pericardial effusion.

Transient Dyspnea: If episodes resolve without intervention, the cause may be transient, such as in pulmonary embolism (PE) or panic attacks.

Recurrent Dyspnea: Ask about past episodes of similar symptoms, as this can indicate a chronic condition such as asthma, CHF, or PE.

Physical Examination

The visual appearance of the patient provides significant clues about their respiratory distress. Some key signs to observe include:

Tripod Position: In severe distress, patients often sit forward with hands on knees, neck extended, and chest propped forward to maximize airway patency.

Retractions or Paradoxical Breathing: These signs indicate mechanical breathing insufficiency, where the chest wall or diaphragm cannot effectively support ventilation.

Grogginess or Lethargy: These symptoms may indicate respiratory fatigue.

Examine the anatomy involved in oxygenation and ventilation, from the airway to the diaphragm and chest wall.

Upper Airway: Dyspnea caused by upper airway obstruction may present with noisy breathing or stridor. Examining the neck using radiographs or contrast-enhanced CT scans can help detect any anatomical obstructions.

Bronchi: Bronchial pathology (e.g., foreign body, infection, or bronchospasm) typically presents with wheezing, which can be confirmed by a chest x-ray showing bronchial cuffing.

Alveolar Pathology: If alveoli are filled with fluid, collapsed, or damaged (e.g., in emphysema), it results in impaired gas exchange and may produce crackles during auscultation. Chest x-rays can reveal consolidations or collapse.

Interstitial Space: Infiltration of the interstitial space with fluid or inflammation leads to decreased oxygen transfer and manifests as dry crackles. Radiographs may show hazy, spongy densities.

Diaphragm: Diaphragmatic dysfunction, due to restrictions like ascites, pregnancy, or muscular paresis, can reduce tidal volume. Asymmetric chest wall expansion on physical exam or abnormal diaphragmatic motion on x-ray can indicate diaphragm involvement.

Chest Wall: Any condition limiting chest wall expansion, such as rib fractures or muscular dysfunction, will result in difficulty breathing. Chest x-rays can identify rib fractures or pulmonary contusions.

Pleural Space: The pleural space, when filled with fluid (e.g., effusion, blood) or air (e.g., pneumothorax), will limit lung expansion, leading to dyspnea. A physical exam may reveal decreased breath sounds or altered resonance, and a chest x-ray or lateral decubitus x-ray can confirm the diagnosis.

Cardiac Considerations

Cardiac dysfunction can also contribute to dyspnea, as it impairs the heart's ability to pump oxygenated blood to tissues. Signs of cardiac involvement can be identified through physical examination, noting murmurs, gallops, or arrhythmias. Cardiac diagnostics should be performed as necessary.

Hemoglobin and Blood Volume

The oxygen-carrying capacity of the blood depends on healthy hemoglobin levels and adequate circulating volume. Conditions like anemia or poisoning (e.g., carbon monoxide) can lead to dyspnea. Assess for signs of anemia, and treat with blood transfusion if required. Ensure adequate blood volume by monitoring vital signs and physical signs like skin turgor and mucous membrane moisture.

Conclusion

Effective management of dyspnea requires a structured approach, starting with identifying life-threatening conditions and working through a differential diagnosis based on anatomical and physiological considerations. A thorough history and physical examination, alongside targeted diagnostic workups, are essential for proper diagnosis and timely intervention.

Suggested Reading

1. Sarko J, Stapczynski S. Respiratory distress. In: Tintinalli JE, Stapczynski JS, Ma OJ, Cline DM, Cydulka RK, Meckler GD, editors. Tintinalli's Emergency Medicine: A Comprehensive Study Guide. 7th ed. New York, NY: McGraw-Hill; 2011. p. 465-473.

Customer Review Request

Thank you for choosing MASTERING CLINICAL EMERGENCY MEDICINE: Core Skills and Strategic Approaches for Fast, Effective Decision-Making. We hope this guide enhances your clinical skills and confidence in emergency settings.

If you found this book helpful, we'd greatly appreciate your honest review on Amazon. Your feedback not only supports other readers in making informed decisions but also helps us continue improving our work.

Thank you for being part of our journey in advancing emergency medicine.

Dr. Joe J. Gaiter & Dr. Johnny S. Lewis

www.ingramcontent.com/pod-product-compliance
Lightning Source LLC
Chambersburg PA
CBHW052346220526
45465CB00003BA/976